Dear Reader:

Expectant parents are quick to fill their shelves with books to prepare them for what's to come. But once the baby arrives, moms and dads want information that's accessible, to the point, and quick to read. We created the *Child* Magazine Guides for just that reason.

What makes this series unique is that each book is intended to help parents of young children deal with a specific problem—fast. The books are written by accomplished journalists who interviewed dozens of leading child psychologists, researchers, and child-care experts and organized their collective wisdom.

If you're a busy parent who needs help *now* to solve the problem featured in this book, I hope you will pick it up and start reading tonight. I'm sure that the small investment of your time will provide a quick return as you implement the solutions we present. Throughout the book, you'll find age flags that will help you easily find the sections that relate most directly to your child.

PAMELA ABRAMS
Editor-in-Chief, *Child* Magazine

Other books in the *Child* Magazine series

Quarreling
Whining
Sleep
Goodbyes
Tantrums

Published by POCKET BOOKS

child Magazine's Guide to

Eating

Win the Food Wars

Ann E. LaForge

A New Century Communications Book

POCKET BOOKS

New York   London   Toronto   Sydney   Tokyo   Singapore

The author of this book is not a physician and the ideas, procedures, and suggestions in this book are not intended as a substitute for the medical advice of a trained health professional. All matters regarding your child's health require medical supervision. Consult your child's physician before adopting the suggestions in this book, as well as about any condition that may require diagnosis or medical attention. The author and publisher disclaim any liability arising directly or indirectly from the use of the book.

An *Original* Publication of POCKET BOOKS

POCKET BOOKS, a division of Simon & Schuster Inc.
1230 Avenue of the Americas, New York, NY 10020

ISBN: 0-671-88041-1

First Pocket Books printing August 1997

10 9 8 7 6 5 4 3 2 1

POCKET and colophon are registered trademarks of
Simon & Schuster Inc.

Cover photo by Tony Stone Images

Printed in the U.S.A.

For Aunt Stevie and Uncle Joe,
who loved and fed me well

Acknowledgments

This book would not have been possible without the generosity of many people. I'd particularly like to thank the following child-care professionals, who donated their time and expertise:

The late Louise Bates Ames, Ph.D., associate director of the Gesell Institute of Human Development in New Haven, Connecticut, and collaborator or coauthor of more than three dozen books, including *The First Five Years of Life, Infant and Child in the Culture of Today* and the series *Your One-Year-Old* through *Your Ten- to Fourteen-Year-Old*

Keith-Thomas Ayoob, Ed.D., R.D., a board-certified pediatric nutritionist, an assistant professor of pediatrics at Albert Einstein College of Medicine in New York City, and director of nutrition services at the Rose F. Kennedy Center at Albert Einstein College of Medicine

Susan M. Bergmann, Ph.D., a child psychologist based in Oakland, California

Felicia Busch, M.P.H., R.D., F.A.D.A., a registered dietitian in private practice in St. Paul, Minnesota, and a spokesperson for The American Dietetic Association, based in Chicago

Rex Forehand, Ph.D., a research professor of clinical psychology and director of the Institute for Behavioral Research at the University of Georgia and a coauthor (with Nicholas Long, Ph.D.) of *Parenting the Strong-Willed Child*

Stephen W. Garber, Ph.D., a behavioral psychologist, director of the Behavioral Institute of Atlanta and coauthor (with Marianne Daniels Garber, Ph.D., and Robyn Freedman Spizman) of a number of parenting books, including *Good Behavior, Monsters Under the Bed and Other Childhood Fears,* and *Beyond Ritalin*

Ann A. Hertzler, Ph.D., R.D., C.H.E., professor and Extension specialist with the Virginia Cooperative Extension at Virginia Tech in Blacksburg, Virginia

Mary Abbott Hess, R.D., L.H.D., F.A.D.A., president of Hess & Hunt Nutrition Communications in Northfield, Illinois, and coauthor of *The Healthy Gourmet Cookbook* and *A Healthy Head Start*

Michael F. Jacobson, Ph.D., executive director of the Center for Science in the Public Interest and a coauthor (with Bruce Maxwell) of *What Are We Feeding Our Kids?*

Sanna James, M.S., R.D., a registered dietitian based in Mill Valley, California, and editor of the newsletter *Tiny Tummies Nutrition News*

Barbara S. Kirschner, M.D., F.A.A.P., a professor of pediatrics and medicine in the Section of Pediatric Gastroenterology, Neurology, Hepatology, and Nutrition at Wyler Children's Hospital in Chicago

Harris Lilienfeld, M.D., F.A.A.P., a pediatrician in private practice in Lawrenceville, New Jersey

Kathy A. Merritt, M.D., F.A.A.P., an associate at Chapel Hill Pediatrics, P.A., in Chapel Hill, North Carolina, and a consulting assistant professor of pediatrics at Duke University Medical Center in Durham, North Carolina

The late Corinne Montandon, Dr.PH., R.D., L.D., an assistant professor of pediatrics and a nutritionist at the Children's Nutrition Research Center at Baylor College of Medicine in Houston, Texas

Carolyn Raab, Ph.D., R.D., L.D., an Extension foods and nutrition specialist at Oregon State University in Corvallis, Oregon

Ellyn Satter, M.S., R.D., C.I.C.S.W., B.C.D., a Madison, Wisconsin-based therapist specializing in the treatment of eating disorders in children and adults, and author of the books *Child of Mine: Feeding with Love and Good Sense, How to Get Your Kid to Eat . . . But Not Too Much,* and the video tape series *Feeding with Love and Good Sense*

Barton D. Schmitt, M.D., F.A.A.P., director of general pediatric consultative services at Children's Hospital of Denver, a professor of pediatrics at the University of Colorado School of Medicine, and author of *Your Child's Health*

Michael Schwartzman, Ph.D., a psychologist in private practice, a consulting psychologist for The Allen-Stevenson School in New York City, and coauthor (with Judith Sachs) of *The Anxious Parent*

Dorothy Sendelbach, M.D., F.A.A.P., an assistant clinical professor of pediatrics at The University of Texas Southwestern Medical Center, in Dallas

Marjorie M. Sutton, M.S., R.D., L.D., C.S., a certified pediatric nutritionist and pediatric nutrition specialist at the University of Chicago Children's Hospital

Carol McD. Wallace, author of *Elbows off the Table, Napkin in the Lap, No Video Games during Dinner*

Ted Williams, M.D., F.A.A.P., a pediatrician based in Dothan, Alabama

Dori Winchell, Ph.D., a psychologist based in Encinitas, California

James Windell, M.A., a clinical psychologist with the Oakland County Juvenile Court Psychological Clinic in Oakland County, Michigan, and author of a number of parenting books, including *Discipline: A Sourcebook of 50 Failsafe Techniques for Parents, 8 Weeks to a Well-Behaved Child,* and *Children Who Say No When You Want Them to Say Yes*

I am also grateful to:

The American Academy of Pediatrics, the American Psychological Association, The American Dietetic Association, the American Heart Association, and the United States Department of Agriculture, for providing background materials and referring me to experts.

The many wise parents who were willing to share with me their concerns and experiences involving children and eating, especially: Carolyn Davenport, Holly DeGregori, Cathy Gilfether, Irene Felsman, Louise Howsmon, Holly Hughes, Monty Hughes, Samantha Hughes, Tekla Jachimiak, Suzanne Koller, Mary Mitchell, Lindsay Monser, Katy Musolino, Rachel Negris, Vicki Nelson, Edie Poole, Julie Ritzer Ross,

Kim Sage, Larry Sienkowicz, Carol Spelman, and Lauren West.

My tireless and inspiring editors, Peggy Schmidt of New Century Communications, Pamela Abrams of *Child* Magazine, and Dave Stern of Pocket Books.

My dear writer friends, who talked me through many a sticky moment, especially Kevin Baker and Gay Walch.

My beautiful children, Gus and Teddy, who unwittingly supplied endless anecdotes and patiently suffered through those last grueling deadline weeks.

My amazing husband Christopher Spelman, whose love and support make everything possible.

Contents

FOUR

*Special Challenges: Coping with a
Picky Eater*

FIVE

*Serious Concerns: Getting a Child to
Eat Less Junk*

Introduction

The Overeater, the Picky Eater, and the Perplexed Parent

My first son, Gus, was a born eater. After six blissful months on breast milk, he made the switch to solid foods and never looked back. He ate everything I ever offered (except raspberries), and he always asked for more.

By the time he was a toddler, Gus could polish off a whole peanut butter-and-jelly sandwich, an entire apple, a handful of carrots, and a cookie—all at one sitting. And he was the neatest eater I've ever seen. Not one crumb fell onto his lap or down to the floor; nary a streak of jam migrated to his hair. He was too intent on making sure *all* the food within his reach made it to his mouth.

I was quite proud of all this, until people started mentioning that my beautiful baby was *fat*. Even my pediatrician seemed concerned when he noticed that Gus was tracking in the fiftieth percentile for height (average) and the *ninety-fifth percentile* for weight (way above average). The doctor didn't actually say I should put my son on a diet, but he did warn me to "watch everything that goes into Gus's mouth." From then on, I watched . . . and worried.

Every time Gus asked for an extra cookie, reached for a french fry, or requested a second serving of snack, my heart sank. I struggled between wanting to say, "Sure, help yourself," and fearing that if I did, he'd end up being a short, overweight, unhappy adult—and I'd be to blame.

It took my second son, Teddy, to cure me of worrying about Gus. Teddy ate at the opposite extreme. From the very start, he fussed and cried during breast and bottle feedings, and he made the switch to solids slowly. I can't remember a food he *liked* before its third or fourth introduction. (Most newcomers to his plate got an unqualified "bleck!") And by the time he was a toddler, his only food groups were peanut butter, cereal, and chocolate milk.

I never worried about Teddy being too fat. Instead, I pictured him as a skinny, scrawny adult with barely enough energy to hold down a job. To prevent this, my husband and I became experts at coaxing for "one more bite." It got to the point where Teddy could pretty much eat anytime, anywhere (on the couch, in his bedroom, in the car), and we'd feel grateful.

It wasn't until I found myself following Teddy around the living room one day, feeding him his lunch bite by bite, that I realized things had gone too far: at the tender age of two, he had learned to use eating to twist me around, like a strand of spaghetti on his toddler-size fork.

That's when I finally stepped back, looked at both of

my healthy, energetic kids, and realized I was on the wrong path with children and food. By worrying too much about *what* my children were eating, I was creating problems in *how* they ate and *how much* they finally consumed.

Feeding Frustrations Are Common

If you have an overeater, a picky eater, or a kid with a knack for turning mealtimes into madness, you probably understand exactly how I felt. And you may be trying all kinds of strategies to improve your child's eating habits—such as withholding junk foods, promising treats if vegetables get eaten, making faces on your child's plate out of sliced fruits, or using funny voices to make healthy foods "talk" (as in: "Hi Alex. I'm Mr. Carrot. I bet you can't eat me!").

If so, don't be embarrassed. There are lots and lots of parents out there who have gone to even greater lengths to make sure their kids eat "right." Some have tried bribing ("If you eat everything on your plate, I'll take you to the park"); some have tried threatening ("If you don't eat your potatoes, you can't play with your new toy"); some have tried begging ("Please, honey, just one more bite of broccoli"). And most, at one point or another, have resorted to yelling ("That's it! I'm tired of listening to you whine for candy. No more candy in this house *ever again!*").

"Eating and nutrition are two of the biggest areas of concern among parents of young children," notes Stephen W. Garber, Ph.D., director of the Behavioral Institute of Atlanta, and coauthor of a number of parenting books, including *Good Behavior* and *Beyond*

Ritalin. "That automatically makes them primary sources of anxiety, frustration, and power struggles."

How It All Begins

For some parents, the trouble begins early, with those first feedings after birth. They expect the image of perfection: new mother, sitting calmly by a window, in a lovely, clean nightgown, smiling serenely as her adorable babe nurses. After all, feeding a baby is supposed to be the most natural thing in the world. But what no one ever tells new parents is that most new babies don't act like the infants in magazine and television ads. Each one has his or her own hunger pattern and feeding quirks, and it often takes a while to settle into an eating routine.

So when reality looks more like this—bleary-eyed mom in rumpled, spit up–stained nightgown, trying to get the nipple into a screaming baby's mouth at two in the morning, wondering why she ever decided to have children; haggard-looking dad standing in the doorway, wondering the same thing—they panic. Then they worry ("Is he eating enough?"; "Is he eating too much?"; "Should we feed him again so soon?"). And all too often, the next step they take is trying to control their child's eating (by waking him up from a sound sleep to attempt a feeding, for example, or making him "cry it out" until the next "scheduled" feeding).

Once a baby's past the milk stage and into solid foods, the questions and doubts begin to multiply. That's because eventually, all children want more say in what they eat and how they eat it. But their ideas of good nutrition and reasonable table manners are a far cry from ours. So even parents whose newborns were easy to feed often start feeling perplexed.

Suddenly their agreeable infant has changed into a baby who spits new foods back in their faces, a toddler who throws terrible tantrums when she can't have a treat, a preschooler who won't eat any foods that are touching each other, or a five-year-old who uses his shirt for a napkin and his fingers as a fork.

Most parents aren't prepared for these behaviors and don't know how to handle them. So again, they attempt to exert control: "Use your fork, Son"; "Don't talk with your mouth full"; "No dessert until you eat your peas"; "Stop kicking your sister"; "Haven't you had enough?"; "Come on now, you *have* to eat something!"

And little by little, the family table becomes a battleground.

Why Do We Worry So Much?

It doesn't have to be that way. "Parents have a tendency to make way too much of what and how their children eat," says Louise Bates Ames, Ph.D., associate director of the Gesell Institute in New Haven, Connecticut. (Dr. Ames was interviewed for this book before her death in 1996.) "They fuss and they force and they fight over these issues, but that usually makes things worse. Most children, if left alone, will eat when they're hungry, stop when they're full, and get all the nutrients they need."

It sounds so easy. So *why* do so many parents have such a hard time "leaving their children alone" when it comes to eating?

There are lots of different reasons. One, of course, is that children exhibit some mighty strange eating behaviors at different stages of development. But even more significant is the fact that we live in a culture that has a love/hate relationship with food. We have access to an incredible array of foods, and we love to indulge our appetites, especially with those high-fat, high-calorie and high-flavor favorites that saturate our environment (fast foods, junk foods, packaged convenience foods, and gourmet desserts). However, we hate the fact that we love those foods, because we now know that eating them can lead to serious medical problems, such as high blood pressure, heart disease, colon cancer, breast cancer, stroke, osteoporosis, and diabetes. Even worse, they contribute to the condition many Americans fear most: overweight.

As a result, we adults have a tendency to classify the things we eat as either "good" (as in good for our health or nonfattening) or "bad" (meaning unhealthy or fattening). We then spend an inordinate amount of time eating, and worrying about what we eat (as in: "How many calories does it have?"; "What's the fat content?"; "Will it make me gain weight?"; "Will it clog up my arteries?"; "Are those additives harmful?"). Or, we don't eat the "bad" foods, and wish that we could ("Those chips look so much better than these carrot sticks"; "The fish tastes fine, but I wish I'd ordered your steak"; "I could kill for a hot fudge sundae").

On top of all that, we have a habit of classifying *ourselves* based on what we eat ("I was so *bad*—I ate the whole bag at once"; "No dessert for me—I'm being *good* today"), and we eat for reasons that have nothing to do with hunger ("I'm so bored; let's go get some ice cream"; "I was so depressed, I ate the brownies"; "Don't start the movie until I make popcorn").

As soon as we have children, of course, we transfer all of our concerns and eating obsessions to them.

"Parents bring a lot more than food into the feeding relationship," notes Corinne Montandon, D.Ph., R.D., an assistant professor of pediatrics at the Children's Nutrition Research Center at Baylor College of Medicine in Houston, Texas. (Dr. Montandon was interviewed before her death in 1997.) "They also bring their own goals, fears, prejudices and emotions about eating. And when those don't match up with their child's behavior, frustration and conflicts occur."

Why and How to End the Conflicts

Ending food conflicts isn't easy, because it requires a parent to acquire new knowledge and a new attitude about food. But it is worth the effort. According to the experts, fussing, forcing, and fighting over eating are the best ways to make any eating-related problem *worse*.

If you really want your child to grow up with a healthy attitude toward food, you need to learn when to get involved and when to let go.

This book is designed to help. Though it does include some information about nutrition, it is not meant to be a guide to feeding. Rather, its focus is the eating behaviors of children from birth to age six, and the eating attitudes of parents that make problems more likely.

Chapter One, for example, looks at the kinds of emotional connections parents often make with food that affect our expectations of what and how our children eat. It also explores what we need to do to break those connections, so we don't mislead our children.

Chapter Two offers a nutritional overview of what kids really need to eat in order to grow and thrive. It puts in perspective both the Recommended Dietary Allowances and the Food Guide Pyramid, using simple language that even a science dropout can understand. And it's broken down into distinct age-related sections, so you can easily focus on the eating stage your child is in.

Chapter Three, which is also divided into age-related sections, explores the developmental, temperamental, and other factors that affect eating behaviors and table manners. Each section features some great discipline tips for the typical, and maddening, eating challenges (food refusals, food jags, and strange food preferences, for instance) that you're likely to face.

Finally, in Chapters Four and Five, you'll get the inside info on the two eating topics that bug parents most: picky eating and junk food.

The research and advice offered throughout this book come from in-depth interviews with more than twenty experts, including registered dieticians, child psychologists, pediatricians, day-care and preschool teachers, and researchers, as well as other parents who know how difficult and ugly family food fights can get. (For a complete list of contributors, see the Acknowledgments.) Their tips and insights may not provide a quick fix for all of your family's food struggles, but they will point you down the best path for raising a child who really eats *right*.

* * *

NOTE: The advice offered in this book is not intended to substitute for the consultation and guidance of the pediatrician, dietician, or other health professional who normally cares for your child. Be sure to call or visit your doctor if you have any questions about your child's diet or health.

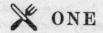

ONE

Emotions: How Caring Can Lead to Overcontrol

"My mom had all kinds of rules about eating when I was growing up," says Lindsay S. Monser, a mother of two. "One was, 'Eat everything on your plate, or no dessert.' So we always ate our dessert on a full stomach. When I got older, I always craved sweets as soon as I felt full.

"Another eating rule was, 'You have to eat at least three bites.' Well, once when I forced down three bites of liver, I ended up throwing it up and crying. And I remember thinking, 'This tastes so gross. Why do I have to eat something so disgusting? Why would my mother force this on me?'

"I know she wasn't trying to be malicious," adds Lindsay. "She had always struggled with her own weight, and she honestly thought that all those rules were necessary to make sure we all ate right. But by the time I was fifteen, I was a compulsive eater, over-weight and unhappy about my relationship with food.

I was a bulemic for three years and a chronic dieter for eight. It took me over ten years to become normal about food, to recover from all the obsessiveness. Now I'm trying my hardest not to let *my* issues and history with food control affect my kids.

"Eating and control," adds Lindsay, "are scary things to mix."

Most eating experts would agree. Yet many well-meaning parents fall into the trap of trying to control their children's eating. They make all sorts of rules about everything from what their children should eat, to when and how they should eat it. Or they coax and cajole and bribe to get vegetables and other healthy foods down their kids' throats. Their intentions are usually good, but the results are mostly dismal.

Not all children end up bulimic, of course. But in the birth-to-age-six range, many cases of overeating, undereating, food refusals, and strange or annoying eating behaviors can be directly traced to parents who care—and control—too much.

That's why the focus of this first chapter is not kids and eating, but parents and their emotions about eating. How you *feel* about food affects what you expect and how you discipline your child when eating issues arise. In addition, how you tend to discipline often determines how extreme your child's eating problems become.

THE THREE MOST IMPORTANT RULES

According to the eating experts, the three healthiest food-related rules you can teach your child are:

1. Eat when you're hungry.
2. Eat a variety of foods from each of the major food groups (including fruits, vegetables, protein, grains, and dairy products).
3. Stop eating when you're full.

That's all your child needs to learn to become an adult who doesn't overeat, doesn't starve herself, and doesn't overconsume the kinds of foods that scientists now say are bad for our health.

It should be easy to instill these guidelines. After all, children are pretty much born with the ability to follow rules one and three. "From the moment of birth, all normal, healthy children have the capacity to regulate their own eating," explains Barbara S. Kirschner, M.D., a professor of pediatrics and medicine at Wyler Children's Hospital in Chicago. "They can tell when they're hungry, they know when they're full, and they can use age-appropriate ways [such as crying or turning away] to let you know which they're feeling."

That means all you have to do is set the table with a balanced variety of foods (which we'll describe in Chapter Two), and leave it at that. Ellyn Satter, M.S., R.D., C.I.C.S.W., B.C.D., a psychotherapist and eating/feeding specialist based in Madison, Wisconsin, refers to this as "the division of responsibility in feeding." In her book *How to Get Your Kid to Eat . . . But Not Too Much*, Satter defines the "golden rule for parenting with food": "Parents are responsible for *what* is presented to eat and the *manner* in which it is presented. Children are responsible for *how much* and even *whether* they eat."

It's Hard to Believe

As logical and simple as this golden rule sounds, many parents have a hard time following it. They just don't buy the part about children knowing when and what to eat. "Most adults have a difficult time regulating what *they* eat," explains Susan M. Bergmann, Ph.D., a child psychologist based in Oakland, California. "So it's hard for them to believe that a child can know when to eat, what to eat, and when to stop."

"Plus, feeding is such a loaded issue for parents," says Dori Winchell, Ph.D., a psychologist based in San Diego, California. "It's not only one of the primary responsibilities of being a parent, it's often viewed as an instant gauge of one's effectiveness as a caregiver. If your child is accepting and enjoying the food you offer, you feel satisfied and competent; but if he's refusing the food or not thriving, you feel like a failure."

This combination of disbelief and vulnerability is a definite handicap when it comes to feeding children. It makes us hypersensitive to all the quirks our kids bring to the table, and more determined to use force when their eating habits seem out of whack (which, since kids don't eat the way adults do, may be most of the time).

The Rules That Don't Work

Typically, when a child's eating seems out of control (for example, he doesn't eat "enough" or he eats "too many" sweets), parents will jump in with a special rule to elicit the behavior they believe is better. For example, to get a picky eater to eat more healthy foods, they might say:

- You have to eat everything on your plate to get dessert.
- You have to clean your plate before you leave the table.
- You can't have sweets before dinner.
- You must eat three square meals a day.
- It's mealtime, so you have to eat whether you're hungry or not.

Parents make these kinds of food rules not because they want to be overbearing and strict, but because, like Lindsay's mother, they want to ensure that their children eat *right*. They want them to be healthy, energetic, and happy. Unfortunately, rules like the ones above usually have the opposite effect. The message they bring to the child is not "Eat when you feel hungry and stop when you're full," but "You can't eat the way your body wants to; you have to eat the way I [the parent] tell you to, because I know best what your body needs."

Unfortunately, that's a dangerous message to send.

"In most cases, when you try to overrule a child's natural eating cues, her eating ends up getting worse, not better," writes Satter. A child who feels forced or tricked into eating, for instance, may end up "revolted by food and prone to avoid eating," she explains. Children who are deprived of or denied certain foods may "become preoccupied with food, afraid they won't get enough to eat and prone to overeat when they get a chance."

Such behaviors tend to increase parental anxiety, of course, and elicit even stronger control tactics; but those only end up encouraging worse and worse eating habits.

The reason is simple: "Young children learn very quickly how to manipulate their parents," explains Mary Abbott Hess, R.D., L.H.D., F.A.D.A., president of Hess & Hunt Nutrition Communications in North-field, Illinois, and a coauthor of *A Healthy Head Start*. "As soon as they see that they can get additional atten-tion for refusing (or overeating) certain foods, they make it their business to create hassles at the dinner table."

The Real Problem

The underlying problem is not that rules are bad for children, or that we shouldn't worry at all about what our kids eat. In fact, there are lots of good reasons why you *should* be concerned about your child's eating hab-its (we'll discuss these in future chapters). And there are appropriate times to set limits on eating behaviors.

"Rules generally protect children," explains James Windell, M.A., a clinical psychologist based in Bloom-field Hills, Michigan, and author of a number of parent-ing books, including *Children Who Say No When You Want Them to Say Yes*. "They give them a sense of security and ensure a sense of order in their life." But that's only if they're used in a consistent, reasonable way.

Unfortunately, Windell adds, many parents use food rules in haphazard ways: to promote their favorite hom-ilies or moral lessons, for example (as in, "A good day starts with a good breakfast"), or to cope with a crisis

("That's it! No more cookies because they always spoil your dinner").

Corinne Montandon, of the Children's Nutrition Research Center at Baylor College of Medicine, agrees. "Parents tend to make eating rules based on their own emotions and eating histories, rather than on nutritional and developmental facts," she notes. "In addition, they're often unaware that they're operating on an emotional level."

EATING AND POSITIVE EMOTIONS

This isn't at all surprising. The temptation to connect eating with emotions is incredibly powerful in our culture. Since we live in a country where food is so plentiful and varied, we have the luxury of viewing it in ways that have nothing to do with physical sustenance. Without even thinking, for example, people frequently use food as:

- *A symbol of love.* My Aunt Stevie and Uncle Joe are perfect examples. I always knew they loved me because every time I visited them, they gave me something wonderful to eat. Sometimes it was candy or cookies; other times it was their mouthwatering corned beef or amazing macaroni and cheese. But what it was never mattered. What did matter was that their kitchen was always warm and cozy, and they always tried to feed me something I liked.

  My great-aunt and great-uncle were following a long tradition. In fact, sharing food is about the oldest, most basic way for one human being to demonstrate care and affection for another. The very act of feeding a child is an act of love, as are:

—cooking a special meal or dessert for someone;

—giving candy on Valentine's Day;

—sending a fruit or gourmet-food basket to a friend or relative who's just had a baby, gotten a promotion, or celebrated an anniversary;

—planning a big feast for a family reunion or holiday celebration involving relatives, coworkers, or friends;

—sharing a piece of wedding cake with a new spouse.

In fact, most of the joyful, love-related occasions in our lives are enriched and enhanced by wonderful foods.

• *A source of comfort.* From the moment each of us first feels the relief of hunger pain from a sip of formula or breast milk, the connection between food and comfort begins. That connection is then reinforced in countless ways:

—when an adult gives a child a cookie after bandaging up a boo-boo;

—when we make a casserole for someone who's sick or grieving; or

—when we take a friend out for a drink because she lost her job or just ended an intimate relationship.

Then, of course, there's chicken soup. "That is probably the ultimate symbol of food as comfort," notes Michael Schwartzman, Ph.D., a New York City–based psychologist, a consulting psychologist for The Allen-Stevenson School in New York City, and a coauthor of *The Anxious Parent*. "As one of my patients once observed, 'There's probably nothing medicinal in the soup. It just makes you feel better because you know there's someone who cares enough to be home cooking it for you.' "

Larry Sienkowicz, a father of two, agrees. "I remember my mother making me a variety of dishes when I was young that made me feel very safe and happy," he explains. "When I was sick, for instance, she'd make me milk toast, which I loved. Or sometimes she'd make me oatmeal or hot chocolate when it was cold out. For some reason, when I ate those foods I felt like I had a mother who wanted me to be warm and cozy and healthy. Even today, I'll sometimes make myself oatmeal or hot chocolate when I want to feel warm and happy. And I make them for my own children now and then, so they can experience those same comforting feelings."

• *An expression of pride and pleasure.* There are lots of good things to eat in our world, so it's no surprise that when people want to treat themselves or celebrate an accomplishment, they often

—go out to a restaurant for a special meal;

—cook exotic foods and share them with friends; or

—splurge on extravagant desserts.

"My parents often used food as a reward," notes mother Julie Ritzer Ross. "When I got a good grade or made the honor roll, for instance, they'd take me out for a celebratory meal. Or, when I was even younger, if I behaved in the supermarket, I'd get a cookie or a doughnut."

"I remember being taken out for ice cream when I got a good report card," echoes Mary Mitchell, a mother of three. "And whenever our family gathered to celebrate a birthday or holiday, there was always a huge feast."

When Positive Emotions Go Awry

Love, comfort, and pride are all positive emotions, and in most cases, there is nothing wrong with connecting them with food—in either your life or your child's. Eating, after all, is one of life's greatest universal pleasures. "However," says Dr. Schwartzman, "problems can emerge if you exaggerate the connection (you *always* use food as a reward or a symbol of love, for instance) or allow your emotions to overrule your child's natural appetite."

Here's the kind of situation you can end up in:

You've just cooked a wonderful meal with all your child's favorite foods, to let him know how much you love him. He comes to the table, takes a few bites, and then asks to be excused because he isn't hungry. You feel hurt and angry because he's not only not eating, he's rejecting your offer of love. So you respond angrily, "I worked hard to cook you that meal. You can't leave the table unless you finish everything on your plate." When he sees how upset you are, he feels guilty, so he makes an attempt to stuff the food down his gullet, even though he's already full. The more he eats, the more his tummy hurts, and the more he resents the way you're manipulating him with food.

The next time you insist that he eat your special meal, he may be hungry, but refuse to eat because he wants to prove that he's the one who's really in charge of his own body. Eventually, the issue of whether or not he's hungry gets lost in the power struggle over who gets to decide when he should or shouldn't eat.

"I remember, as a child, being forced to taste certain foods," recalls Monty Hughes, a father of two. "But then I wouldn't eat them no matter what, even if I liked the taste or felt really hungry, because I was determined not to be forced."

Here's another example: Say you always reach for a high-fat, high-calorie, or sugary food when you want to comfort your child, or show her you're proud of her ("After I put on the Band-Aid, we can have some cookies and milk"; "You did a great job behaving in the store; now let's get ice cream"). Eventually, like Pavlov's dog, she's going to connect one with the other—and every time she does something well, she'll crave a treat.

That may not be a big problem when she's a child, but when she gets a little older and her calorie and nutrient needs change, it's likely to lead to weight and health problems.

"That's what happened to me," says parent Julie Ritzer Ross. "The connection between food and reward became so strong that I would routinely reward myself with an ice cream sundae or some other food treat when I passed a test or got a good grade. By the time I was in high school, I had a serious weight (and self-esteem) problem that took years of dieting to overcome."

Avoiding Problems

Anytime you feel personally hurt or rejected by your child's eating behaviors or preferences, it's a good sign that you're overmixing eating and emotions—and you need to pull back. As Windell notes, "When parents start saying or implying things like 'If you loved me, you'd finish all of it' or 'I've tried so hard to cook a meal you'd like, and you can't even sit at the table and eat it,' they are encouraging the kind of excessive guilt that causes children to be anxious and dependent. They are not encouraging good eating habits."

———————————— ✳ ————————————

Worksheet #1:
Parent Checkup: How Often Do I Use Food to . . .

(Circle Your Response)

Show my child I love her	Never	Sometimes	A Lot
Help my child feel better when she's hurt or sad	Never	Sometimes	A Lot
Show my child I'm proud of him	Never	Sometimes	A Lot

If you circled "A Lot" for any of the above, try to think of at least two nonfood ways that you could:

Show your child you love her	1. _____ 2. _____
Give your child comfort	1. _____ 2. _____
Express pride and pleasure in his accomplishments	1. _____ 2. _____

Now try to use these techniques, rather than food, the next time the issues of love, comfort, or pride arise.

———————————— ✳ ————————————

EATING AND NEGATIVE EMOTIONS

When it comes to negative emotions, the one that gets most parents in trouble when feeding children is fear.

What do parents fear most about food? The two primary concerns are:

1. *Fears about getting fat.* This is probably the biggest fear most Americans—especially women—have in connection with eating. We have it because we live in a culture that's constantly throwing out mixed messages about eating and weight. On the one hand, our environment is saturated with tempting foods that add little more than calories and flavor to our diet. On the other hand, we're constantly bombarded with media images that insist that the perfect way for a woman to look is like a teenage boy with breasts (no hips, no butt, no stomach), and to be a real man, you've got to have clearly defined biceps and hard-as-rock abs.

"Plus," notes Dr. Bergmann, "there are all sorts of moral values placed on eating." For instance, many people believe that if you're overweight, it must mean that you can't resist the temptation to eat "bad" things, so you must be a "bad" person; if you're thin, it must mean that you're somehow "good."

"For a woman, in particular, eating 'too much' is often associated with shame and guilt," adds Dr. Bergmann, "and there's a lot of fear that if you start eating everything you want, you won't be able to stop."

The result is a billion-dollar diet industry, and a huge percentage of the population who feel unhappy about how much they weigh, how much they wish they could eat, and how their bodies look.

As one parent I interviewed admits, "I can't remember a time when I didn't worry about my weight. I went on my first diet when I was ten, and I've been going on and off them ever since. It's been a terrible struggle, and no matter how thin I get, I never feel like the battle is over.

"I'd do anything to save my child from the misery of dieting," she adds.

Most parents would—and many try to. In fact, one recent study, published in *Pediatrics*, found that approximately 40 percent of 9- and 10-year-old American girls were trying to lose weight; for most of them, the dieting had been triggered by a comment about their weight from their mothers.

"A lot of women who are struggling with their own weight become overly concerned about their children's weight, too," notes Felicia Busch, R.D., M.P.H., a registered dietitian in Saint Paul, Minnesota, and a spokesperson for The American Dietetic Association (ADA). "Their basic feeling is, 'It happened to me and it was awful, so I'm never going to let it happen to you.'"

2. *Fears about getting sick.* Unless you've been living in a secluded monastery for the past few years (which is highly unlikely if you have kids), you're probably well aware of the fact that diet is now considered a significant risk factor in a number of serious medical conditions, including heart disease, stroke, high blood pressure, colon and breast cancers, osteoporosis, obesity, and diabetes. This news has had a definite dampening effect on how many Americans view food. Now we have to worry not only about how many calories we take in, but how much fat, saturated fat, cholesterol, and sodium we consume. The fact that all

of these play major roles in the foods we tend to love and crave only makes life a little more difficult.

The research findings linking diet to disease in adulthood have also raised concerns about children's diets: If we're at risk, won't they be, too? Shouldn't we teach them now to avoid the foods we're having such a hard time giving up as adults? Those are the kinds of questions scientists *and* parents are now asking. And although the complete answers aren't yet in, many parents aren't taking any chances. Even if they haven't been entirely successful at changing their own diets, they're determined to make sure their children eat healthy. So they count every gram of fat, sugar, cholesterol, and sodium that goes into their kids' mouths.

On the other end of the scale are the parents who fear that their picky eater isn't eating enough. These parents worry about things like stunted growth, malnutrition, and diminished brain power. As parent Larry Sienkowicz puts it, "Sometimes when I sit at the table and watch my three-year-old take two bites of bread, one bite of vegetables, and no bites of meat, I feel certain that he'll end up being a malnourished pipsqueak with an underdeveloped brain. I can't help worrying about what he eats."

When Our Fears Take Over

Is that so bad? Shouldn't all parents be concerned about their child's weight and health? "Of course," says Windell. "But there's a big difference between concern and overconcern." Concern is when you take the time to learn about how children grow and develop and how their development affects their eating; then you offer your child foods that are appropriate to her age and health.

Overconcern is when you start imposing eating rules based on your desire to *save* your child from the kind of eating mistakes you've made, *protect* him from the fears you harbor, or *shape* his body (through under-feeding or overfeeding) to fit the ideal image in your mind. Those are the behaviors that put a child right in the path of trouble.

Again, it's that problem of eating mixed with too much emotion: the more caught up you are in your own anxieties about weight and health, the more likely you are to get overinvolved in what your child eats. In addition to imposing strict rules, you may end up:

• Spending a great deal of time talking and arguing with your spouse about what your child should or shouldn't be eating ("He's had way too much candy today"; "I think he should eat his squash before he gets dessert!"; "You can see he's getting fat and you still feed him all that junk"), or making comments about your child's appearance or weight ("You're getting a little pudgy, there, Son");

• Becoming overzealous about teaching your child what is and isn't healthy (as in, "You can't have that, honey, because it's full of fat and fat is bad for your heart," or "If you don't eat more food, you're going to stop growing");

• Forbidding your child to participate in certain activities and outings (such as going to amusement parks, birthday parties, friends' homes, or fast-food restaurants) because he'd end up eating unhealthy foods;

• Attempting to bribe your child into eating certain

healthy or low-calorie foods (as in, "Zoom! Zoom!
Here's the zucchini plane. It's heading straight for
your mouth. Open up!" or "If you want to have a
frozen yogurt pop after dinner, you have to eat all of
your potatoes");

- Religiously counting the fat and calories in what your
child eats, to make sure she sticks to the same low-
fat, low-calorie regimen you're trying to suffer
through;

- Feeling and acting like you're a failure at parenting
because you couldn't get your child to eat a "good"
breakfast; you gave in to his whining for a candy bar;
you've had to resort to hot dogs and chips for supper
more than once this week; or you're too tired to come
up with another creative strategy for getting your kid
to eat vegetables;

- Modeling a distorted eating pattern by serving your
child or other family members balanced meals while
you pick at a salad every night, or by depriving yourself of sweets all week and then loading up on doughnuts, steak, and soda pop all weekend;

- Putting your child on a diet.

Good Intentions, Bad Results

As well-intentioned as all of these actions may be, they
don't produce the desired results. Instead of teaching
children to avoid the kinds of negative food habits that
encourage excess weight gain, and the kinds of foods
that put a body at risk of disease, they demonstrate that
food can be used as an emotional hot button. They
overemphasize the importance of appearance over
health, they discourage eating out of hunger, and they

encourage children to crave (and sneak) forbidden foods. Most of all, they link food to negative emotions such as shame, guilt, and fear, instead of connecting it to hunger.

"Anytime you make your child feel bad or guilty about wanting or enjoying certain foods, you open the door to even bigger eating problems like bulimia, anorexia, and obesity," says Ted Williams, M.D., a pediatrician in Dothan, Alabama. And most children are having a hard enough time as it is, he adds. "I've been a pediatrician for twenty years, and I've never seen boys and girls as worried about their body image as they are today," he adds. "With all the emphasis on health, fitness, and dieting, children are finding it tougher to believe that it's alright to look 'okay.' They think their bodies have to be perfect—so they're eating and dieting in all kinds of unhealthy ways."

You probably won't face body-image problems in the birth-to-age-six years, he adds, but what you say and how you act when you feed your child now will definitely have an impact on how your child feels about food and eating later on.

Worksheet #2:
Parent Checkup: Am I Overanxious about What My Child Eats?

(Circle Your Response)

I talk about food in front of
my child   Never   Sometimes   A Lot

I argue with my spouse about what my child should eat	Never	Sometimes	A Lot
I won't let my child eat certain foods because they're either too unhealthy or too fattening	Never	Sometimes	A Lot
I worry aloud about my own diet and health	Never	Sometimes	A Lot
I won't serve dessert unless other foods are eaten first	Never	Sometimes	A Lot
I use games and tricks to get my child to eat fruits and vegetables	Never	Sometimes	A Lot
I won't let my child eat any foods that are high in fat	Never	Sometimes	A Lot
I won't let my child eat candy or other foods that are high in sugar	Never	Sometimes	A Lot
The food I eat is often different (i.e., less fattening) from what I serve my child	Never	Sometimes	A Lot

The more times you circled "A Lot," the more you need to reexamine your fears and anxieties about food. Be sure to read Chapters Two and Three, to get a clearer perspective on normal eating needs and behaviors in early childhood.

———————— ✳ ————————

YOUR EATING HISTORY

Now that you've gotten a glimpse of how parental
emotions can undermine a child's natural eating pattern—and encourage the kinds of eating behaviors
you'd dearly love to end—it's time to take a look at
what *you* bring to the table.

"All parents bring a certain amount of emotional
baggage into the feeding relationship," notes Windell.
"The table manners, food rules, and eating myths you
grew up with all influence how you approach feeding
your child."

They can also determine how you discipline your
child when eating problems emerge. For example, say
your three-year-old refuses to eat meat. You think she
should eat it for her own good, so you start trying to
trick her or force her into eating it (as in, "If you take
a bite of meat, you can have a bite of cookie" or "No
Teddy Bear Grahams until all your meat is gone"). The
more she resists, the more anxious and angry you get,
until every meal becomes a battle over meat.

Instead of focusing on how you can get your child to
eat meat, you should be asking yourself:

1. Why is it so important to me that my child eats
   meat? and
2. Is my expectation of my child realistic, based on her
   age and stage of development?

"A lot of times, when it comes to expectations about
what a child should eat or how she should behave at
the table, parents operate on autopilot," notes Dr.
Bergmann. "They do what their parents did, without

thinking about whether or not the old rules make sense, or whether their child is actually old enough to be able to comply. That's why it's so important to define the fears behind your food rules. Once you look at your concerns in the light of day, you can usually see whether or not they're rational."

For example, if you're reflecting on why you want your child to eat meat, you may suddenly remember that your parents had a strict rule about eating meat at every meal, and you hated it. You may also remember that nutritionists no longer believe that meat and potatoes at every meal is a healthy way to eat. You can then calm your fears by telling yourself, "Meat was considered an important dietary element in my parents' generation. Nowadays, however, meat is not considered so important. There are other foods that can supply my child with the protein she needs. Instead of fighting with my child over meat, I'll just make sure I serve other protein-rich foods that she enjoys."

Uncovering Hidden Conflicts

In some cases, as you examine your motives for forcing a certain kind of food into your child's mouth, you may discover that your real source of stress has nothing to do with the food or your child's reaction to it. "For some parents, the underlying problem is that they're feeling out of control in some other aspect of their life: for example, work is going badly or they've just had a fight with their best friend or spouse," notes Dr. Stephen Garber, of the Behavioral Institute in Atlanta. "Or it may turn out that they're feeling threatened by their child's growing independence. Because they feel out of control, they impose food rules on their kids to gain a sense of control over something."

"I definitely think that was behind some of my mother's strict food rules," says parent Lindsay Monser. "As a stay-at-home mom with four kids to care for, she was under a tremendous amount of stress. She felt powerless in her position as a housewife and mother, yet she had all this responsibility to raise her kids 'right.' Controlling what we ate was one of the ways she helped herself feel in control."

If you can get to the heart of your emotions, you can often pull away from needless struggles over food and concentrate on fixing what really needs to be fixed. Instead of yelling at your child to eat more meat, for instance, you may need to get more child-care support from your spouse, talk to your boss about your workload, or apologize to your friend.

Untangling your emotions won't always be easy. As Dr. Schwartzman points out, "There are usually many troubling elements going on at once in every situation involving food and feeding. But there is generally one central issue that makes a person feel close to losing control. It's important to try and stay with your anxiety a moment, and listen to what's really causing you to feel deflated, upset, or tense when a food-related power struggle occurs."

Sorting Out the Facts

It's also important to collect the factual information that will enable you to decide whether or not your concerns are worth fighting over. As nutritionist Montandon notes, "The more you learn about nutrition and child development, the better prepared you'll be for the normal—but annoying—food preferences children show at different ages."

If you know that picky eating is common in the toddler and preschool stages, for instance, then you won't panic when your two-year-old suddenly decides to eat only once a day, or your three-year-old dissolves into tears because her favorite food is touching something else on her plate. Instead, you'll be able to stay calm and tell yourself, "This is normal behavior. It will not put my child at any health risks. If I don't make a big deal out of it, this behavior will eventually go away." Or, when your five-year-old rejects the feast you've prepared in her honor, you won't think "She's rejecting me," you'll be able to tell yourself, "Oh well, I guess she's just not hungry right now."

At the same time, you'll feel more confident about taking action if your six-year-old refuses to eat anything from her lunch box besides Hawaiian Punch and Skittles, or your one-year-old gets in the habit of throwing food at the wall.

In the next few chapters, you're going to find a lot of information about what children need to eat to stay healthy, and when you should—and shouldn't—worry about your child's diet. You'll also learn more about how eating behaviors shift and change as children grow and develop, and how best to respond to the various feeding challenges your child dishes out. This information will serve as your reality check as you sort out your emotional reactions to your child's eating behaviors.

In the Meantime . . .

Anytime you start feeling anxious or angry about what, how, or how much your child is eating, your first reaction should be to examine your own eating history and emotions. Then you should compare your child's behavior with the current thinking on child development and nutrition. "That way," notes Dr. Schwartzman, "you'll be better able to determine whether your food-related concern is realistic, or you're loading the scene with a lot of inappropriate emotion."

Worksheets Three and Four in this chapter are designed to help you with the process of reflection. Try to find a quiet moment to complete both of them before you continue with this book. And make sure your spouse or other significant caregiver in your child's life fills them out, too. If your memories and expectations about eating are radically different from your partner's, you're going to need to work at finding some common ground. As Windell points out, "Parenting is always more effective when the adults in charge are on the same wavelength."

※

Worksheet #3:
Parent Checkup: How Was I Raised to View Food?

The following questions are designed to help you remember what eating was like in your childhood home. Take a moment to review them, and then jot down your answers on a separate piece of paper. Ask your partner or other significant caregivers in your child's life to do the same. Then, take some time to sit down and discuss the similarities and differences in how you were raised to view food. Try to agree on the attitudes and discipline methods you'd like to either continue or avoid as you feed your own children.

1. What is my earliest memory of food or eating? What is the strongest emotion I connect with that memory?

2. What was a typical family meal like in my household? (For example: Who was there? Where did you eat? What kind of food was served? What was the conversation like? What was the overall mood of your parents and siblings? How did you usually feel when the meal was over?)

3. What were some of our most predictable mealtime routines? (Did you always eat at the same time every day? Did you usually eat as a family? Did the menu vary much day to day? Did you always say grace?)

4. What kinds of eating behaviors did my parents get most upset about? What were their main eating-related rules, and how did they enforce them? Did I think they were being fair?

5. Which of my parents' food-related rules would I like to pass on to my own child? Why?

6. Which of my parents' food-related rules am I determined to avoid with my own child, and why?

7. What was my typical reaction when new foods (or foods I didn't like) were served? How did my parents usually respond?

8. What did I enjoy most about eating with my family?

9. What did I enjoy least?

10. What do I consider my biggest hang-ups about food and eating?

11. Did my parents ever comment on my weight, appearance, or health? If so, what kinds of comments did they usually make, and how did they make me feel?

12. How do I feel now about my weight and appear-

ance? How concerned am I about my diet and my
health?

———————————— ✳ ————————————

———————————— ✳ ————————————

Worksheet #4:
Parent Checkup: What Worries Me Most about My Child's Eating Habits?

You probably wouldn't be reading this book if you
didn't have some strong worries, doubts, or other emotions about what, how, or how much your child is eating.
This worksheet is designed to help you define your concerns, so you can put them into clearer perspective as
you read this book and learn more about nutritional
needs and developmental stages.

A. What are the three things that worry me most about
   what, how, or how much my child eats? (For example:
   "He never eats" or "He never stays seated at the
   table.")

   1. _____

   2. _____

   3. _____

B. What are my deepest fears about what will happen if
   I can't get these behaviors to stop? (For example:
   "He'll end up malnourished" or "I'll get so angry, I'll
   slap him.")

   1. _____

   2. _____

3. _____

C. What words best describe the atmosphere during most of our family meals? (For example: pleasant, chaotic, boring.)

_____ _____ _____

_____ _____ _____

D. What would I most like to change about our family meals?

_____

_____

_____

——————————— ✳ ———————————

——————————— ✳ ———————————

Six Positive Ways to Influence Eating

Children aren't born with eating habits intact. "They learn which foods to eat, how much to eat, and when to eat as they interact with the people around them," explains Carolyn Raab, Ph.D., R.D., L.D., an Extension foods and nutrition specialist at Oregon State University in Corvallis. Parents, in particular, she adds, can wield enormous influence simply by playing six key roles:

1. *Gatekeeper.* Most children will do whatever they can to influence food purchases. But you hold the ultimate power to decide which foods make it into your home. Use that power to expose your child to a variety of nutritious foods.

2. *Role model.* Though researchers aren't yet certain how young children develop food preferences, many believe that imitation plays a key role. "A mother who eats salad and drinks diet soda all day is sending an unspoken message about eating to her child," notes Raab. "So is a father who says, 'I hate peas—don't serve me any.' "

3. *Stage manager.* Research shows that criticism, conflict, and stress at the dinner table lead to poor diets and play a part in eating disorders. But a pleasant mealtime atmosphere can set the stage for healthy eating habits. "It's up to parents to make meals a time for relaxed family interaction," says Raab.

4. *Director.* This involves establishing a reliable schedule for meals and snacks, and making sure your expectations of what your child will eat and how she'll eat it (in her high chair, with a spoon, with a bib, etc.) are realistic. That way, her appetite won't be destroyed by frustration.

5. *Teacher.* Informal conversations about the kinds of food that promote good growth and health can take place anytime, anywhere: in the grocery store, in front of the TV, or at the dinner table, for instance. You can also cultivate an interest in good foods by teaching your child to help choose and prepare it.

6. *Mediator.* Children are constantly bombarded with misleading ads about food and health. "Parents can lessen the impact of advertising by pointing out the difference between commercials and TV shows, and explaining that advertising sells foods by making them sound as appealing as possible," Raab says.

❋

✕ TWO

Nutrition: What Kids Really Need to Eat

It was one of those days. No matter what I put in front of Teddy (then two), he wouldn't eat. He played with his food. He dropped carrots on the floor. He pushed apple slices off his plate. But as far as I could tell, very little was reaching his mouth.

By the time he announced "I done," my fears were confirmed: All he had eaten were three bites of sandwich, two apple slices, and five out of ten raisins.

I was certain that wasn't enough. "There must be *something* else I can get him to eat!" I told myself as I scoured the cupboards for one more food to offer.

"Aha!" I said, finally, fishing out a snack from the back of the shelf. "How about a granola bar, Teddy?"

He clapped his hands, his eyes sparkled and he smiled broadly as he reached for the treat. But two bites later, he was out of his high chair and on his knees, playing with his train set; the granola bar was left in the dust.

Still, I wasn't ready to give up. I picked up the sticky snack bar and knelt down next to my son, trying to convince him to finish it.

Lunch lasted about two hours that day.

If I knew then what I know now, that scene (and many others like it) would never have happened. Instead of worrying that my son was starving himself, I would have cleared his plate and thought to myself, "Not bad. He had some sandwich, some apples, and some raisins." Then I would have left the kitchen and joined him and his Thomas train for some fun at the tracks.

But back then, like many parents I had no clear idea of what kids really need to eat to survive. Nor was I certain how to react when meals did or didn't get eaten. As a result, I was constantly second-guessing myself: "Is he eating too much?"; "Is he eating too little?" And I was easy prey for all the well-meaning people who said things like, "You should feed him more vegetables"; "He's too skinny"; "All that sugar will make him hyperactive"; and "I can see his rib cage—are you sure he's getting enough to eat?"

Breaking the Pattern

According to the experts, I'm not alone. "I see many parents going to one of two extremes," notes Harris Lilienfeld, M.D., F.A.A.P., a pediatrician in Lawrenceville, New Jersey. "They either worry too little and let their kids consume massive amounts of junk food, or they worry too much and place unnecessary and often harmful restrictions on what their children eat."

Both patterns are destructive, he adds. But there is a

way to break them: become informed. The more you understand about human nutrition and how it applies to young bodies, the less you'll worry when your kid's plate comes back barely touched, or he starts asking for seconds and thirds of foods you fear are fattening or bad for his health.

You don't need a degree in nutrition to qualify as an informed parent. Nor do you need to obsessively count the grams and calories in your child's food to feel confident you're serving nutritious fare (who has time for all that, anyway?). All that's required is a basic familiarity with:

- The nutrients that are most important to a growing child's body;
- The food groups that supply the different nutrients; and
- The amount of food it actually takes to satisfy a child's nutritional needs at different ages.

This chapter will review the basics for you. It is not intended to be a complete guide to childhood nutrition, but a general introduction to some of the major nutritional concepts involving kids from birth through age six. The finer points—when *your baby* is ready to switch formulas or start solids, for instance, or what you should serve *him* for breakfast—should be worked out between you, your pediatrician, and your child.

———————— ✳ ————————

Analyzing Food Claims

Dietary fads are rampant these days and hard to resist. "When you care so much about your child's health and development, it's easy to get caught up in the excitement of a new diet or vitamin supplement that promises better weight control, health, or longevity," notes nutritionist Felicia Busch. "But the research still shows that variety and balance are the most important elements in a child's diet."

So before you put your child on any nutritional bandwagons, ask:

1. *Does this food claim sound too good to be true?* If so, it probably is. There is no scientific evidence that any one particular diet, herb, vitamin, mineral, enzyme, or food can cure or prevent any illness. Diet is but one of many factors that affect a person's health and life span. Changing what you eat can reduce your risk for certain diseases, but it cannot completely protect you (or your child) from a specific illness.

2. *Is the claim backed up by carefully controlled experiments?* If not, look before you leap. Personal anecdotes and testimonials can be very persuasive, but what works for one person doesn't necessarily work for another. In most cases, if the medical community is not behind a new food fad, it's either because the claim is considered unsafe or there's no evidence that it actually works for most people.

3. *Would following this claim involve restricting variety in my child's diet?* If so, reject it. As Busch notes, "As soon as you start restricting or overpromoting specific foods or ingredients (even healthful ones), you undermine your child's ability to get the proper mix of nutrients."

———————— ✳ ————————

1   THE BASICS

AGE FLAG: BIRTH AND UP

WHAT EVERYONE NEEDS

The first step in creating a sensible diet for your child is understanding what the human body requires from food to survive. Here's a quick overview:

The Role of Nutrients

When we chew and swallow food, our bodies immediately begin breaking it down into distinct, minute substances known as nutrients. This process continues as the food travels through the gastrointestinal tract, from the mouth to the stomach, and on to the small intestine. Once the nutrients have been sufficiently separated, they pass into the bloodstream and begin supplying our individual cells with the substances they need to thrive.

Different nutrients perform different jobs, so our bodies need all of them to run smoothly. But there are six that are particularly important to people of all ages.

The Essential Nutrients	What They Do
1. Proteins	Help the body build, repair, and replace tissues; contribute to the production of hormones, enzymes, and antibodies; aid in the transportation of nutrients and oxygen throughout the body; can act

	as a source of energy if carbohydrate supplies run low.
2. Carbohydrates	Supply most of the energy that enables the body to process other nutrients, maintain normal bodily functions, and fuel physical activity.
3. Fats (or lipids)	Provide energy; supply fatty acids, which are necessary for proper growth and functioning; aid in absorption of vitamins A and D; make food more flavorful and filling.
4. Vitamins	Enable the body to operate smoothly. Among the most important in childhood are:
Vitamin A	Plays an important role in vision; helps protect mucous membranes; promotes growth and resistance to infections.
Vitamin D	Enables the body to absorb and use calcium and phosphorus to build strong bones and teeth.
Vitamin C	Helps the body maintain healthy bones, teeth, skin, and tendons; heal wounds; resist infection; absorb iron.
B Vitamins	Control the use of carbohydrates and help the body perform various other vital functions.

5. Minerals	Aid in the regulation of nerve responses, muscle contractions, and electrolyte balance. Among the most important in childhood are:
Calcium	Builds strong bones and teeth; enables heart and other muscles to contract; helps blood clot.
Phosphorus	Aids calcium in building strong bones and teeth; enables heart and other muscles to contract.
Iron	Helps produce hemoglobin, a protein that carries oxygen in the blood to the body's cells.
Fluoride	Prevents dental cavities; strengthens bones.
6. Water	Carries nutrients and oxygen through the body via the blood and lymphatic systems; helps maintain bodily temperature; removes metabolic wastes through urine and sweat; lubricates joints; maintains most life-sustaining chemical reactions.

* * * * ✳ * * * *

Other Important Elements

In addition to the essential nutrients, our bodies need an assortment of other dietary substances to operate smoothly. Two important examples are:

1. *Fiber*

This term refers to a variety of substances in plant foods that have no nutritive value and cannot be digested, but:

- Add bulk to the stool and help prevent constipation;
- Protect against gastrointestinal disorders;
- Reduce blood cholesterol (which may reduce the risk of cancer, cardiovascular disease, and diabetes later in life); and
- Create a feeling of fullness that discourages overeating and obesity.

It's important to look for ways to add fiber to your child's diet. According to The American Dietetic Association (ADA), based in Chicago, "Children in the U.S. are not getting enough dietary fiber to promote health and prevent disease."

2. *Calories*

A calorie is a unit of measure that reflects the fuel or energy value of different foods. We all need to consume a certain number of calories each day, to maintain an adequate weight and fuel our growth and bodily functions. We get most of our calories from carbohydrates, proteins, and fat. Alcohol is also a source of calories. Fat, however, is the most concentrated source (with nine calories per gram, instead of the usual four).

When we take in too few calories, we lose weight and our bodies begin burning protein from our muscles for energy; if we take in too many calories, the extras are converted into fat, which causes a gain in weight.

Because they are active and growing, children generally need more calories, pound for pound, than do adults. A twenty-nine-pound toddler, for instance, needs about 1,300 calories; and a forty-four-pound five-year-old needs about 1,800. In comparison, the average 140-pound adult woman with a desk job needs about 2,000.

At any age, the most healthful caloric intake is one that provides an individual with just enough energy—not too much, not too little—to maintain a healthy weight and sustain bodily functions. Fortunately, our bodies are quite good at telling us what we need (although as adults we don't always listen). If your child is allowed to honor his internal cues—to eat when he's hungry and stop when he's full—he'll get the perfect amount of calories for his needs.

THE RECOMMENDED DIETARY ALLOWANCES

While children and adults require the same combination of nutrients to survive, they need them in different amounts. That's why the Food and Nutrition Board of the National Academy of Sciences–National Research Council regularly updates a list of the daily protein, calorie, vitamin, and mineral needs of people at different ages. This list is known as the Recommended Dietary Allowances (RDAs). The RDAs are based on an ongoing review of research involving the nutrient requirements of people around the world. They vary according to age and sex, and there are special categories for women who are pregnant or nursing.

The RDAs for each nutrient are given in scientific measurements such as grams, micrograms, milligrams, and equivalents. In general, they are set high, to compensate for the various rates at which different individuals absorb nutrients.

While it's important to be aware of the RDAs and the nutrients they cover, it is not necessary to memorize the numbers, routinely calculate your child's nutrient consumption, or panic if her intake seems inadequate on any given day.

Like most of us adults, children feel hungrier on some days than on others, and they eat different amounts at different meals. If they don't consume the RDA of protein on Monday, for example, they're likely to eat more than they need on Wednesday or Friday. Usually, over the course of a week it all balances out.

As nutrition expert Mary Abbott Hess notes, "Good nutrition is about food, not numbers. If your child eats a variety of healthful foods, you don't have to worry about the numbers."

2   FEEDING INFANTS

AGE FLAG: BIRTH TO 6 MONTHS

How Infants Get Their RDAs

From a purely *nutritional* standpoint, there's nothing easier than feeding a baby. That's because a new mother's body comes prestocked with the perfect food for a human infant: breast milk. And for women who can't or don't want to breast-feed, there are a number of commercially made formulas that do the trick nicely.

BREAST MILK

The Perfect Food

If you choose to breast-feed, you'll find that breast milk is the ideal source of nutrition for your baby during her first six months of life. "I'm a big fan of breast-feeding, even if a mother can't do it full-time, or can only do it for a short time," notes Keith-Thomas Ayoob, Ed.D., R.D., a board-certified pediatric nutritionist and director of nutrition services at the Rose F. Kennedy Center at Albert Einstein College of Medicine in New York City. "It's full of all the right nutrients in all the right amounts."

"Plus, there are a number of ingredients in human breast milk that technology [and cows] cannot reproduce," adds Dr. Ayoob. And the human breast does something that no other food source can: It constantly alters the composition of its milk to meet a baby's changing needs.

At first, for instance, the breasts produce colostrum, a thickish, yellow fluid that provides a newborn with water and sugar, as well as fat, protein, minerals, and white blood cells (which protect the infant's health). There is no artificial substitute for colostrum, which is why many experts recommend that even women who plan to formula-feed their babies try to breast-feed for at least the first few days or weeks of life.

After about three to five days of colostrum, the breasts begin producing a thin, bluish-looking milk. But the quantity and quality of this milk keep evolving. For instance, at the beginning of a feeding, the breasts supply a watery "fore milk," which appears to satisfy the baby's thirst and desire to suck; after a while, a richer "hind milk" comes in to fill and nourish the infant. Breast milk also adjusts itself according to the baby's age, growth rate, and appetite.

Additional Advantages

There are other nutritional advantages to breast milk, according to Dr. Ayoob:

- It's easier for babies to digest (and therefore less likely to cause colic, gas, or excessive spitting up than cow's milk or formula);
- It contains less sodium and protein than cow's milk, and thus is easier on a baby's developing kidneys;
- It enhances the absorption of calcium;
- It rarely causes constipation or diarrhea;
- It is rarely the source of a food allergy;
- It contains important antibodies that bolster a baby's immunity to colds, ear infections, and other illnesses.

What It Doesn't Provide

The only two nutrients breast milk does not provide are vitamin D and fluoride, but both can be easily obtained.

Most light-skinned full-term infants get adequate vitamin D from normal sun exposure; however, preterm infants, babies who get less than fifteen minutes of sun exposure a day, and dark-skinned infants may need a supplement. (Ask your pediatrician.)

To cover fluoride needs, many pediatricians prescribe a supplement for breast-fed babies, to prevent later tooth decay. This supplement can be discontinued as soon as your baby begins consuming four to eight ounces of water a day (if your local water supply contains fluoride).

Depending on how long you breast-feed, your pediatrician may also recommend an iron supplement for your child. Breast milk has relatively low supplies of iron. And while most babies are born with a stockpile of iron reserves, their supplies tend to run out by around four to six months of age. Unless you've started your child on an iron-fortified cereal by then, a supplement may be necessary. An iron deficiency in the first year and a half of life can cause serious developmental and behavioral problems.

How Much Is Enough?

One of the beauties of breast-feeding is that you don't have to worry about quantity. As Dr. Lilienfeld puts it, "If Nature wanted you to worry about volume, your breast would be transparent and there'd be a gauge on it." As long as you feed your baby on demand (whenever he cries to be fed), and he seems to be thriving, you're giving him the perfect amount. In addition, the more he nurses, the more milk your breasts will produce, so there's little chance that your supply will fall short of his demand, even when he goes through a growth spurt. (For more on demand feeding, see Chapter Three.)

✳

Eating for Two

If you're breast-feeding your baby, your diet is as important as hers is, according to Corinne Montandon. To produce quality breast milk, you must increase your usual intake of *calories*—by about 400 to 500 a day. But that doesn't mean you should go hog-wild with hamburgers, doughnuts, and chocolate cake. Instead, strive for a daily intake of:

* six to eleven servings of breads, cereals, pastas, rice, and other grains;
* two to three servings of meat, poultry, fish, beans, eggs, or nuts;
* two or three servings of milk, yogurt, cheese, or other dairy products;
* two to four servings of fruits;
* three to five servings of vegetables;
* two quarts of fluid (milk, juice, water).

(You'll need even more of these healthy foods if you're nursing more than one baby or are a vegan.)

In addition, your doctor may prescribe a multivitamin to make sure you get enough vitamin D, calcium, and phosphorous.

One more thing: Certain foods a mother eats can affect how her baby feels. For instance, some breast-fed babies react negatively to the milk and other dairy products their mothers eat. "If your baby has explosive stools or streaks of blood in his stool, you should call your doctor," advises Dr. Barbara Kirschner. Otherwise, trial and error will help you see which foods to avoid while breast-feeding.

Also, be sure to go easy on the alcohol, and avoid any drugs that don't carry the blessing of your doctor.

———————————— ✳ ————————————

COMMERCIAL FORMULAS

The Next Best Thing to Mother Nature

If you are unable or unwilling to breast-feed, or you would like to supplement your breast-feedings with a bottle, the best choice—nutritionwise—is a commercial, iron-fortified infant formula. "Infant formulas are a safe alternative to breast milk," notes Barton D. Schmitt, M.D., F.A.A.P., a professor of pediatrics at the University of Colorado School of Medicine, and author of *Your Child's Health*. "Bottle-fed babies grow as rapidly and are as happy as breast-fed babies. And a special advantage of bottle feeding is that the father can participate."

Different Choices

The infant formulas available today are not quite perfect substitutes for breast milk. For one thing, there is no equivalent for colostrum. In addition, formula has neither the easy digestibility of human milk nor the protective antibodies. However, formula does appear to provide all of the energy and nutrients a healthy, full-term infant needs.

This wasn't always the case. The earliest forms of commercial infant formula generally consisted of whole or evaporated cow's milk mixed with sugar and water. The protein levels in those early formulas were much higher than what's found in human milk; the fat was largely saturated, poorly absorbed, and deficient in essential fatty acids; the carbohydrates consisted of both lactose and sucrose.

Though most of today's commercial infant formulas are still derived from cow's milk, they've been significantly modified to resemble breast milk more closely. For instance, the protein content has been reduced, the butterfat has been replaced by animal–vegetable fat mixtures, and only lactose (not sucrose) is now added.

Infant formulas are also now fortified with iron and other essential nutrients to ensure well-rounded nourishment.

For infants who are allergic to the protein in cow's milk, or who for other reasons can't tolerate a cow's milk-based formula, there are two other options:

- *Soy-based formulas*—which are made with soy protein and have no lactose; and
- *Protein hydrolysate formulas*—which are mainly designed for infants who can't tolerate formulas from either cow's milk or a soy base. (However, because of their lower-quality taste and higher cost, these formulas are usually recommended only for babies with allergies to cow- and soy-based formulas, or with other severe feeding problems.)

"Most infants do well with cow's-milk formulas, and those are generally the first choice among pediatricians," notes Dr. Lilienfeld. "However, if you notice any symptoms of food intolerance—such as vomiting, diarrhea, significant constipation, rash, or, in extreme cases, problems with swelling, breathing, or swallowing—within thirty minutes of a bottle feeding, you should consult your doctor about switching to another type of formula."

Proper Preparation

Most commercial infant formulas come in three forms: powder, concentrated liquid, and ready-to-serve liquid. Although they vary in price and convenience, their nutritional value is more or less equal. However, if you use either the powder or the concentrated liquid forms, it is *extremely important* to follow the measuring and mixing instructions on the package.

"New parents are sometimes tempted to try and save money by adding more water than specified when mixing a batch of formula," notes Kathy A. Merritt, M.D., F.A.A.P., an associate at Chapel Hill Pediatrics P.A., in Chapel Hill, North Carolina, and a consulting assistant professor of pediatrics at Duke University Medical Center in Durham, North Carolina. "Others think that by adding more powder or concentrate, or less water, they're creating a 'richer' drink for their child." But making infant formula is not like making chocolate milk, says Dr. Merritt. With the latter, adding a little extra fluid or powder mainly alters the taste; with infant formula, it alters the amount of calories and nutrition the baby receives.

If you dilute the formula, for instance, your baby will have to drink more to get the calories she needs. This will not only stretch her stomach capacity, it can be harmful. Excessive fluid intake can cause brain swelling, lethargy, or seizures in an infant. If you serve a too-concentrated version of formula, your baby will get more calories than she needs and may end up gaining unnecessary weight.

So, unless your pediatrician specifically advises otherwise, always stick to the package directions and use accurate measuring utensils when mixing your baby's brew.

How Much Is Enough?

Some parents feel more comfortable using formula instead of breast milk because they can tell exactly how much their baby is drinking. That's all fine and good, as long as you don't get too caught up in the numbers. If you try to force your newborn to drink a specific amount, or eat according to a strict timetable, you'll both end up frustrated and unhappy, and you'll hamper your baby's ability to follow her inborn hunger and fullness cues. (For more on how much to feed, see Chapter Three.)

------------------------- ✳ -------------------------

Please Don't Pass the Milk—Yet

If most infant formulas are derived from cow's milk, why not just use the real thing?

It sounds logical. But the American Academy of Pediatrics (AAP) and others involved in infant nutrition strongly recommend *not using* any form of cow's milk during the first *twelve months* of life. That includes not only whole, skim, one-percent, and two-percent milk, but powdered milk (which becomes skim milk when mixed with water) and evaporated milk (which becomes whole milk when mixed with water).

According to the AAP, the disadvantages are many. For instance, cow's milk:

* Is difficult for a human baby to digest;
* Contains very little iron, and therefore puts an infant at risk of iron deficiency;
* Has much higher levels of salt and protein than either breast milk or formula, which can strain an infant's developing kidneys;
* Has too little zinc and vitamins A, C, and E, and too

much protein, calcium, and phosphorus to support a baby's rapid growth and development;
* Is linked to a higher incidence of milk allergy than either formula or breast milk.

3 FEEDING BABIES

AGE FLAG: 4 TO 6 MONTHS

HOW BABIES GET THEIR RDAS

If breast- and/or bottle feeding is going well, there is no need to add anything to your child's diet until he's about four to six months old. After six months, however, he'll need more than milk alone can provide.

SOLID FOODS

When to Begin

You'll probably hear a lot of conflicting advice about when to start your baby on solids. One reason is that the idea of feeding a baby nothing but liquids for up to six months doesn't make sense to most adults. We equate liquid diets with deprivation and fasting or weight-loss diets. But to most babies, drinking breast milk or formula is the next best thing to being back in the womb. They get everything they need—cuddling, comfort, satiety, and nutrients—from bottle or breast.

Another reason is that the guidelines for spoon feeding have been all over the map in recent generations.

Back in the early 1900s, for example, when sanitation and refrigeration of foods were still iffy, the rule was to keep a baby on breast milk only, for the first year. In the 1930s, when vitamins were discovered, solids were suggested at four to six months, to ensure adequate nutrition. From there, the trend moved toward earlier and earlier feedings, mainly because babies seemed to accept them. By the mid-1950s, some experts were recommending starting solids by the third *day* of life and cutting out nighttime milk feedings when an infant was about two weeks old.

The pendulum, however, has swung back to a more moderate level. "Nowadays, most pediatricians recommend starting solids sometime between four and six months of age, with six months being the optimum," according to pediatrician Dr. Ted Williams. The reason for this has more to do with development than nutrition.

Developmental Factors

Although perfectly designed for sucking, newborns have no natural flair for eating solids. They're born with something called an extrusion reflex, which causes the tongue to push anything even remotely solid out of the mouth. As one nutrition expert points out, "To get a spoonful of baby food within swallowing range of an infant under four months old, you literally have to push the spoon to the back of the baby's throat, which forces her to gag and swallow reflexively."

The extrusion reflex usually fades around the third or fourth month of life. But it isn't until four to six months of age that the typical baby starts needing more calories than she can get from a full tummy of milk. At that point, you can either add on extra milk feedings (or—God forbid!—resume previously abandoned night feedings) to up the supply of calories, or (the better choice) introduce a more concentrated source of energy: solids.

Signs of Readiness

Since development is more important than age when it comes to starting solids, your pediatrician will want to look at a number of factors before giving you the go-ahead. These include not only how much your child is drinking and how well he's growing, but how well he can:

- Swallow;
- Sit upright in an infant seat or high chair and control his head and neck;
- Recognize a spoon;
- Open and close his mouth;
- Reach out or lean forward to show his interest in food when others are eating or food is nearby;
- Turn his head away or lean back to show he's full or not interested in what you're offering.

If your child has not reached these milestones, or appears to be developmentally delayed, your pediatrician may advise you to wait a while before wielding a spoon. The final decision, of course, is up to you. But it's worthwhile to remember that spoon feeding too soon will increase frustration, not nutrition.

How to Begin

Once it's clear that you and your baby are ready to move beyond the milk diet, the name of the game is to start slowly. "There is no nutritional or other reason to hurry your child into trying new foods," notes Dr. Lilienfeld. "It should take about six more months before your baby is getting two-thirds of her nutrients from food and only one-third from formula or breast milk."

According to the AAP, the best strategy for early feedings is to offer *one (very liquidy) food at a time, at intervals of a week or more.* This will not only enable your baby to get used to each new food at a comfortable pace, but allow you to quickly identify the source of any adverse food reactions.

While the sequence of food introductions is not critical, most pediatricians recommend starting with a pre-cooked, single-grain infant cereal (usually rice, barley, or oatmeal) that's been fortified with iron. These cereals are a good first choice because they are usually well-tolerated and they add iron to the diet just around the time the baby's own stores are becoming depleted. Plus, you can mix these cereals with either breast milk or formula to create a more familiar flavor.

From baby cereal, you can move on to thin purees of individual vegetables (such as carrots, green beans, or yellow squash), and then to nonacidic pureed fruits (such as apples, pears, or bananas); the last step should be meat and eggs.

Keeping Things Pure

Each new food should be presented in its pure form—in other words, without any of the added sugar, salt, butter, cream, spices, or other seasonings we adults usually depend on. A baby's taste buds aren't yet trained to require the extra flavorings, and those ingredients may place an unnecessary burden on your baby's developing digestive system and kidneys. Plus, if you salt, season, or sweeten a food, or add gravy or sauce, and then your child has a reaction to the food, it will be more difficult to identify the culprit: Was it the vegetable or something in the cream sauce?

This is especially important if you, your spouse, or other family members suffer from food allergies (a trait that can be passed along to a child), or your child appears to be allergy prone (he already has asthma or eczema, for instance). "In high-risk children (see box, page 52), the onset of allergies can sometimes be delayed by being extra careful about their diet," notes Dr. Schmitt.

Even if your baby is not at high risk for food allergies, if she shows any of the following reactions within three or four days of trying a new food, you should immediately stop offering it:

• Excessive bloating or gas;
• Diarrhea;
• Mucus in the stool;
• Vomiting;
• A rash around the mouth or anus;
• Runny nose and/or watery eyes;
• Wheezing;
• Unusual crankiness;
• Nighttime wakefulness.

You can reintroduce the food after about a week, but if a similar reaction occurs, withdraw the food and consult your pediatrician.

❋

Understanding Food Allergies

Food allergies are a big concern among parents of young children, but according to Dr. Schmitt, they tend to be overdiagnosed. "Only about five percent of children have true reactions to food," he says, "and many of those affected have a family history of food allergies."

Still, it's better to be safe than sorry. You should suspect a food allergy, says Dr. Schmitt, if your child has the following *combination* of symptoms:

1. Swelling, diarrhea, hives, or difficulty breathing or swallowing after eating certain foods (among infants, eggs and milk products are the most common culprits; in older children, peanuts, peanut butter, soybeans, soy formula, wheat products, fish, shellfish, and tree nuts are the most common triggers);
2. Problems with other allergic conditions, such as eczema, asthma, or hay fever;
3. A parent or sibling with diagnosed food allergies (risk is highest if both parents have them).

If a food allergy is suspected, you should consult your pediatrician. If it's confirmed, you'll need to eliminate the offending food from your child's diet. If an entire food group is involved, the doctor will probably prescribe a supplement.

"The good news," adds Dr. Schmitt, "is that at least half of the children who develop a food allergy during the first year of life outgrow it by age two or three."

❋

How Much Is Enough?

You'll probably be surprised at how little your baby needs to eat during early spoon feedings:

- With first introductions, the general guideline is *one or two teaspoons*, served on a tiny baby spoon, of course.
- Once your child gets going with a food, you can gradually increase the serving size to about *two to four tablespoons*.

But babies vary, so you need to read your own child's cues. Whatever you serve, the trick is to start out small. The main course at each meal is still breast milk or formula; the pureed food is there mainly to whet your baby's appetite for learning more about eating, and to increase her intake of calories.

How to Progress

Sometime around eight to ten months of age, your baby will be ready for more frequent solid-food meals and will settle into a pattern of eating that roughly corresponds to your breakfast, lunch, and dinner. She'll also begin to consume more varied meals, with mixtures of different foods: a little cereal and some fruit for breakfast, for instance, or a bowl of vegetables and a little meat for lunch. And once her teeth begin popping out, she'll be ready for a variety of finger foods: bite-size pieces of soft foods (such as cubes of cooked carrots, soft cheese, or bread; soft crackers; or individual pieces of cooked pasta or dry cereal).

"As you see this progression evolving, you should start thinking about variety in your child's diet," advises Dr. Kirschner. In addition to at least two cups of breast milk or formula, an older baby's daily menu should include:

- *Fruit and vegetables*, including some rich sources of vitamins A and C (such as applesauce, spinach, yellow squash, and sweet potato) and iron (such as pureed broccoli or kale);
- *Grains* (such as iron-enriched baby cereal, crackers, pasta, and bread);
- *Protein* (meat, fish, poultry, cheese, beans, legumes, eggs).

Do not, however, expect your child to eat his fill of each of the above food categories at every meal, or on every day. Some days he may concentrate on vegetables; other days on fruit. But if you keep offering a variety of foods, it will all add up to a balanced diet.

Choke Alert

Never feed your baby any of the following, since they may cause choking:

- nuts (especially peanuts)
- hard, round candies
- chewing gum
- whole grapes
- whole olives
- whole cherries or other pitted fruits

* popcorn or corn kernels
* sunflower seeds
* raw carrots, celery, or green pepper
* cubes of hard cheese
* hot dogs

When Should You Add Juice?

The easiest answer to this question is: as soon as your baby starts learning to drink from a cup (which, for most kids, means around six to eight months old). You can, of course, serve juice in a bottle. But saving it for the cup works as a nice incentive for your baby to move beyond the bottle.

The best choice is a one hundred-percent-fruit juice (avoid juice drinks with lots of sugar in them), and it's a good idea to dilute the juice with water, according to Dr. Williams. (Full-strength juice is full of natural sugars.)

While juice does provide carbohydrates and vitamin C for a baby, and most babies love it (even when it's cut with water), it is not the nutritional equivalent of breast milk or formula. So it's important to offer no more than seven or eight ounces a day. "Any more than that may kill your baby's appetite for the nutrient-rich milk on which her body still depends," Dr. Williams adds.

Water should also be offered from a cup or bottle, especially on hot days, when your baby is in a dry environment for extended periods, or when he has a fever.

4   FEEDING TODDLERS

AGE FLAG: 1 TO 2 YEARS

How Toddlers Get Their RDAs

By the time your baby celebrates her first birthday, she should be ready to join the family in a regular mealtime routine. You can pull her high chair right up to the table and serve her modified versions of whatever everyone else is eating (assuming you're all consuming a varied, healthful diet).

Important Modifications

Switching to Cow's Milk

Much to the relief of everyone who thought you should have switched your baby to cow's milk months ago, you now have the official go-ahead. Your baby's digestive system is more mature and better able to handle the protein and other substances in cow's milk, and the bulk of her nutrition is now coming from food.

"There is, however, still one restriction," notes Dr. Kirschner. "You should *not* serve skim or low-fat (one-percent or two-percent) milk just yet." Your baby still needs the fat contained in whole milk to develop cushions around nerve endings and sustain other vital growth.

Most one-year-olds need about two cups of milk a day. This amount not only provides your child with good amounts of vitamins A and D and protein, it confers a generous gift of calcium. Toddlers and older children need lots of calcium (about 800 milligrams a day) to build good, strong bones and teeth, and keep their muscles working and their blood clotting. While most dairy products (i.e., cheese, yogurt, and ice cream) supply calcium, milk is about the best source because it has so much: about 280 milligrams per eight-ounce cup.

"If your child rejects milk, it's important to find other ways to supply his calcium requirements," notes Extension specialist Carolyn Raab. Yogurt and cheese are generally the next best sources, but he can also get calcium from:

- Dishes made with milk or powdered milk, such as puddings, soups, mashed potatoes, scrambled eggs, pancakes, breakfast cereals, vegetables with cheese sauce, ice cream, milkshakes, or cocoa;
- Canned fish, such as sardines, anchovies, and salmon;
- Dark green leafy vegetables such as kale, mustard greens, and turnip greens;
- Tofu (processed with calcium sulfate);
- Orange juice fortified with calcium;
- Lactose-free milk; and
- Tortillas made from lime-processed corn.

If your child shows an extreme sensitivity or allergy to milk and milk products, or is diagnosed with a lactose intolerance, you may need to switch to a fortified soy milk or a lactose-free brand (such as LactAid); your doctor may also recommend calcium supplements.

Store-Bought Versus Home-Cooked

Deciding between commercial toddler foods and home-cooked meals is a matter of cost and convenience, not nutrition. If you find it more convenient to buy specially packaged toddler foods, feel free to do so. Otherwise, just about anything you prepare at home can be offered to your child. (The one exception? You're better off with an iron-fortified baby cereal than with a box of sugar-laden regular cereal, since your baby still needs lots of iron.)

How Much Is Enough?

The best rule of thumb for serving sizes, from now until your child is about eight years old, is to offer *one tablespoon of each food for every year of your child's life*. If your child is one, and you only put one tablespoon of chopped chicken and one tablespoon of soft-cooked carrots on her plate, with half a slice of whole-wheat bread, you aren't starving her. You're giving her portion sizes she can deal with. If she eats everything and seems satisfied, you'll know she's had enough; if she wants or needs more, you can happily serve it; and if she only picks at her food or just ignores it, you can assume she doesn't want or need that particular food at that particular meal.

Scheduling in Snacks

You should count on your child needing snacks, says Montandon. Unlike adults, children don't have large enough stomachs to make it through the day on three meals. They need frequent small meals and snacks to sustain their high energy levels and keep their bodies growing.

The trick is to make sure the snacks are spaced so they don't interfere with mealtime hunger. They should also be viewed as part of your child's overall daily nutrition package, not as sugary or salty treats to punctuate the day. As Montandon notes, "Since young children have such tiny tummies and such big nutrition needs, every bite they take counts."

What about Vitamins?

This is an age when many parents truly feel their child is living on air and that vitamin supplements are the only way to ensure proper nutrition. But many pediatricians and nutritionists don't agree. As Dr. Schmitt notes, "In our society, vitamins tend to be overused. And contrary to popular myths, they do not improve a child's appetite, prevent infections, or increase pep and energy. In some cases, in fact, (namely with vitamins A and D) if they're taken in excess, they can build up in the body and cause headaches, kidney stones, and other health problems."

"If your child consumes a regular balanced diet and eats food from all of the different food groups," adds Dr. Schmitt, "he'll be fine."

On the other hand, if your child is an extremely picky eater and is failing to grow properly, or has a restricted diet for a specific medical reason, vitamin supplements may be helpful or necessary. While it's best to make the decision to use or not use them with your pediatrician, if you do decide to strike out on your own, make sure:

• Any vitamin supplement you give your child is specially formulated for a person your child's age—not for an adult;
• You never give more than the recommended dose;
• You keep all vitamin supplements out of reach, so your child won't feel tempted to sneak a dose on her own (in excess, vitamins and minerals—especially iron—can be toxic).

———————— ✳ ————————

Vegetarian Kids

Can kids survive without meat? Definitely. But if you want your child to be a vegetarian, you should take certain precautions:

Birth to Twelve Months

• If possible, choose breast-feeding over a soy formula for the first six months.
• Let your pediatrician know of your plans to raise a vegetarian; ask about vitamin supplements to ensure adequate intake of iron, vitamins B and D, and folic acid.

Twelve Months and Up

• Avoid a true vegan diet (the kind with no meat, fish, poultry, eggs, milk, and other dairy products) while your child is under age two. As Hess points out, "Without dairy products, children cannot get enough calcium for bones and teeth, nor iron for red blood cells, and may not get enough calories to meet basic energy needs." These deficiencies can affect brain growth.

- Offer only whole-grain beans and cereals to your toddler, to supply the vitamins, minerals, and proteins he won't be getting from meat and other animal sources.
- Offer a variety of protein-rich foods each day, along with tofu and other soy-based products;
- When using nuts, whole grains, and seeds, make sure they are sufficiently ground or chopped to prevent choking.
- If your child won't be consuming milk or other dairy products, make sure she gets plenty of calcium from other sources (tofu prepared with calcium, broccoli, and other green leafy vegetables, finely ground almonds, and pine nuts, for instance); ask your pediatrician about a calcium supplement.
- Serve lots of iron-rich foods (such as legumes, whole-wheat bread, leafy green vegetables, and fortified breakfast cereals) and include vitamin C at every meal to enhance iron absorption.
- Don't go overboard in restricting high-fat foods such as oils, nuts, seeds, and butter, since these provide lots of calories;
- Ask your pediatrician about a vitamin supplement to give your child sufficient amounts of iron, zinc and vitamin B12 (which are difficult to obtain for children who don't eat meat, fish, or poultry).

5 FEEDING BIG KIDS

AGE FLAG: 2 TO 6 YEARS

HOW BIG KIDS GET THEIR RDAS

By the time your child is two, he's officially ready to follow the official "Dietary Guidelines for Americans" issued by the U.S. Department of Agriculture (USDA) and the U.S. Department of Health and Human Services. These are the same guidelines we adults are supposed to follow to ensure that we meet our RDAs. The main difference is that kids need fewer servings.

The Dietary Guidelines do not stray far from the advice already given for kids under age two. Updated in 1995, they describe a pattern of food choices designed to "help Americans choose diets that will meet nutrient requirements, promote health, support active lives, and reduce chronic disease risks." In general, they take the moderate path.

Not everyone in the nutrition world is happy with the Dietary Guidelines (some people think they're too lenient about red meat and animal fats, for example, while others believe they're too strict). But for the purposes of directing a huge, diverse population through a controversial field in which no one yet knows all the answers, they're a good start. They are most helpful if you use them as a map, not as a rule book.

Here's how to tailor the Dietary Guidelines to kids:

Guideline #1: Serve a Variety of Foods

As mentioned before, it takes a little of this and a little of that to create a balanced diet. There are two key ways to guarantee variety in your child's diet. One is:

• *Serve some food from each food group every day.*

Remember those essential nutrients we talked about at the beginning of this chapter? While all of them are found in varying amounts in different foods, specific

groups of food (commonly known as food groups) provide either more or more-efficient forms of different
nutrients. Just check out the chart below.

———————————————— ✳ ————————————————

The Food Group	What It Includes (Some Typical Foods)	What It Provides (Major Nutrients)
1. The grain group	Bread, cereal, rice, pasta, crackers, bagels, muffins, rice cakes	Carbohydrates Vitamins Iron Fiber
2. The vegetable group	Raw or cooked vegetables; vegetable juice and soup	Carbohydrates Vitamins (A and C) Minerals Fiber
3. The fruit group	Raw or cooked fruits; fruit juice	Carbohydrates Vitamins (A and C) Minerals Fiber
4. The milk group	Low-fat milk, yogurt, cheese, custard, ice milk, pudding	Vitamin D Calcium Protein Fats
5. The meat and beans group	Lean meats, poultry, fish, dried beans and peas, tofu, eggs, peanut butter, cold cuts	Protein Iron Fats
6. The fat group	Butter, oils, margarine, mayonnaise, sweets and treats	Fats

———————————————— ✳ ————————————————

Each of the above food groups is represented in
the USDA's Food Guide Pyramid, which is a visual

tool designed to help people follow the Dietary Guidelines. Also included in the pyramid are recommended serving sizes—or how much a person should consume from each food group over the course of a day to meet RDAs. The number of servings per day for children is, naturally, smaller than what's recommended for adults. But the serving sizes themselves are also smaller, so don't panic when you first look at the numbers in the chart below, from the USDA. Often a child will eat more than one official serving at a meal (one cup of milk, for instance, represents two servings) and more than satisfy her nutrient requirements.

Sample Food Choice Pattern for children aged two to six:

The Food Group	Number of Servings/Day	Approximate Size of One Child-Size Serving
The grain group	4–6	• 1/2 to 1 slice bread • 1/3 cup rice, pasta, or hot cereal • 2/3 oz. cold cereal • 4 small or 2 large crackers
The vegetable group	3	• 2/3 cup leafy raw vegetables • 5 tbsp. cooked vegetables • 1/3 cup chopped raw vegetables • 1/2 cup vegetable juice • 2/3 cup vegetable soup
The fruit group	2	• 1 small piece of fruit • 1/2 large piece of fruit • 1/3 cup berries • 1/3 cup canned fruit • 1/2 cup fruit juice

The milk group	4	• 1/2 cup milk • 3/4 to 1 oz. cheese • 1/2 cup yogurt
The meat and beans group	2–3	• 1–1/2 to 2 oz. cooked lean meat, poultry, or fish • 1 egg • 1/2 cup beans • 2 tbsp. peanut butter

✳

The very tip top of the Food Guide Pyramid represents the fat group. This basically includes butter, oils, margarines, and other sources of animal fat, as well as most sweets and treats—candy, cakes, cookies, ice cream, chips, dips—you name it. There is no official serving size for this group, but only a piece of to-the-point advice: *use sparingly.* Or, to put it more directly: Don't use fats unless you really need to.

More Variations

The second most important strategy for ensuring variety in your child's diet is:

• *Serve a variety of foods from within each food group.*

"In other words, if your child loves fresh fruit, don't just relax and keep offering bananas and apples every day," says Busch. "That will limit her taste buds and her nutrient intake." Instead, help her expand her palate with strawberries, melons, raspberries, mango, kiwi, and other fruits. Each different type of fruit will supply a different combination of vitamins and minerals. For instance, oranges, plums, and raisins are all considered fruit. But while oranges are a great source of vitamin C, plums offer a generous boost of vitamin A, and raisins contribute to iron stores.

"Serving a variety of foods within each food group makes it even more likely that your child will get everything she needs, nutritionwise," notes Corinne Montandon. That, in turn, will make your job easier, since you won't have to sweat the details of her daily diet. You'll know that if she doesn't finish her vegetables, she'll still be able to meet her vitamin and mineral needs with fruit; if she hates meat, she can still get adequate protein from beans and eggs; if she refuses milk, she can still get calcium from cheese or yogurt.

Guideline #2: Serve Plenty of Grain Products, Vegetables, and Fruits

These foods are pictured at the base of the Food Guide Pyramid to underscore the idea that they provide the strongest foundation for a healthy diet.

This wasn't always the prevailing belief. A generation ago, the foods in these three food groups—salad, baked potatoes, rice, pasta, mixed vegetables, and fruit cup, for instance—were viewed mainly as appetizers or side dishes to a big piece of meat. But today, nutritionists are urging people to treat them as focal points of the meal, with an occasional small piece of meat on the side.

There are a few logical reasons for this:

• Grain products, vegetables, and fruits are chockful of essential vitamins, minerals, complex carbohydrates, and other substances vital to good health;

- They are great sources of dietary fiber, which not only improves digestion and bowel function, but may help lower the risk of cancer and heart disease;
- They are rich in antioxidants, such as beta-carotene and vitamin C, which appear to confer protection from cancer, and phytochemicals (plant chemicals, such as flavonoids and isoflavones), which may protect against tumors;
- Unlike red meat, grains, fruits, and vegetables are low in fat (unless you cook or serve them in fat, of course), so you can eat your fill without worrying that you're overdoing the fat group.

Even so, most Americans of all ages eat far fewer than the recommended number of servings of grains, vegetables, and fruit. In one USDA survey of elementary school kids, only thirty percent had eaten a piece of fruit that day; according to a National Cancer Institute study, one in four children eats less than one serving of vegetables a day. So if you aren't already doing so, it's worth it to pay more attention to these food groups when feeding your child.

———————— ✳ ————————

Easy Changes: Adding Fruit, Vegetables, and Grains

- Serve your child four to six servings from the grain group each day.
- Choose products made with whole grains (such as wheat, oats, corn, millet, buckwheat, and barley) instead of processed grains (white bread or white rice) whenever possible.

- A few times a week, make beans, peas, or lentils the main attraction of a meal instead of meat.
- Offer at least one fruit and one vegetable at every meal. (What's wrong with a carrot at breakfast?)
- Favor dark green leafy and deep yellow vegetables, which are jam-packed with important vitamins.
- Prepare and serve vegetables with little or no fat (such as salad dressing, butter, or cream sauce).
- Serve fresh fruits as desserts and snacks.
- When preparing one-pot meals or casseroles, increase the amount of vegetables and decrease the amount of meat in the recipe.

Guideline #3: Serve Foods That Are Low in Fat, Saturated Fat, and Cholesterol

By now, just about everyone knows that fat and cholesterol are the biggest bad guys in the American diet. Widely publicized studies have linked them to heart disease, stroke, obesity, and certain forms of cancer. The average American adult has been warned many times over to reduce daily fat intake to no more than thirty percent of calories, and many experts believe less would be even better.

But, what's good for adults is not always good for children. As mentioned in previous sections, children under age two need a lot of fat to grow and develop properly. If you reduce your child's fat intake too soon, it may hamper development of her vital organs, such as the liver, spleen, kidneys, and brain. "Even modest dietary changes—such as switching from whole milk to two percent milk—are *not advised* for babies and children under two," notes Montandon.

Once your child has passed her second birthday, however, you should begin to think about gradually lowering the fat in her diet. Before, when she was growing rapidly but eating smaller amounts of food, she needed the extra calories in fat to fuel her growth. Now, however, her growth rate is slowing down. Plus, she's eating a greater quantity and variety of foods, so it's easier for her to get all the calories and nutrients she needs from lower-fat sources.

Still, there's no reason to go overboard on fat reduction. If you severely restrict fat intake, or attempt to eliminate fat entirely from your child's diet, you will put your child at risk of vitamin deficiencies, growth problems, and poor health. A more reasonable goal, according to the Dietary Guidelines, is to gradually shape your child's diet so that she's consuming no more than thirty percent of total calories from fat by the time she's about five years old.

For a two- or three-year-old who's consuming about 1,300 calories a day, the thirty percent fat mark translates to about forty-three grams of fat per day; for a four- to six-year-old who's eating 1,800 calories a day, the grand total would be sixty grams of fat.

The Fats to Avoid

Even more important than limiting total fat is reducing the amount of saturated fat your child eats. Dietary fats come in two basic varieties: saturated and unsaturated. The former is called saturated because its fat molecules are drenched with hydrogen atoms. This type of fat is considered undesirable because studies have shown that a high consumption of saturated fat raises the level of low-density lipoprotein (LDL) cholesterol in the blood.

Lipoproteins carry tiny clusters of cholesterol, fat, and protein through the blood. LDLs are considered bad because they tend to leave the cholesterol stuck to the interior of artery walls, causing heart-threatening blockages over time. High-density lipoproteins (HDL) are considered good because they carry cholesterol down to the liver and out of the body.

Keep in mind that some foods and food groups can contain more than one type of fat.

Saturated fat is mainly found in such oils as coconut, palm kernel, and palm, as well as in dairy products, meat, and poultry. The experts say saturated fat should account for no more than ten percent of your child's total calories each day, but most American kids consume much more.

Unsaturated fats do not increase blood cholesterol, and are therefore favored over their saturated counterparts. They come in two versions:

• *polyunsaturated fats*, which are found mainly in corn, cottonseed, safflower, soybean, and sunflower oil, as well as in some types of fish, margarine, mayonnaise, and nuts; and
• *monounsaturated fats*, which come in olive and canola oils, chicken, shortening, meats, and dairy products.

Although it doesn't appear to raise the risk of heart disease, unsaturated fat should still be eaten "sparingly": it is high in calories and, like saturated fat, may increase cancer risk.

If you start reading the Nutrition Facts Labels on foods, you'll notice that many of the most popular packaged kids' foods also contain something called *partially hydrogenated vegetable oil*. This basically means that the oil in the food has been mixed with hydrogen to make it more solid (as in margarine sticks and vegetable shortening). Unfortunately, it also means that there's more saturated fat and something called *trans fats* in the product. Although technically unsaturated, trans fats are known to raise blood cholesterol, and are therefore considered just as undesirable as plain old saturated fat.

Dietary Cholesterol

In addition to fat, *dietary cholesterol* should be a concern, especially if you have a family history of heart attack, angina, stroke, or bypass surgery. Dietary cholesterol is found only in animal-related foods such as poultry, meat, eggs, fish, and dairy products, but in some people it plays a significant role in raising blood cholesterol. In others, it appears to have very little effect. No one knows for certain why this is, but genetics may play a role.

Studies have shown that high blood cholesterol levels in childhood tend to translate to high levels in adulthood. So, according to the AAP and the American Heart Association, if there is a history of high blood cholesterol in your family, your child's cholesterol levels should be measured after age two, and periodically monitored. If the levels are high, your doctor may put your child on a special program of diet and exercise.

Even if you don't have a family history of heart disease, it won't hurt to try and lower the cholesterol in your child's diet, just to be safe. Most American children consume far more than they need.

✳

Easy Changes: Reducing Fat and Cholesterol After Age Two

* Switch from whole milk to one percent or skim milk.
* Instead of ice cream, serve low-fat or fat-free frozen yogurt.
* Choose low-fat cheeses.
* Cut down on hot dogs, hamburgers, sausages, bacon, bologna, and other luncheon meats; when you do serve them, choose the low-fat, extra-lean, or vegetarian varieties.
* Trim fat from meat and remove skin from chicken before serving.
* Use less fat and oil when cooking; avoid frying.
* Avoid foods made with palm and palm kernel oil, coconut oil, cocoa butter, hydrogenated vegetable fat or shortening, lard and partially hydrogenated fats.
* When you use ingredients like salad dressing, butter, margarine, and mayonnaise, use smaller than usual amounts or buy the low-fat or fat-free versions.
* Read food labels and choose snacks and lunch foods that are lower in saturated and hydrogenated fats.
* Season vegetables and other foods with herbs, spices, lemon juice, and fat-free or low-fat dressings instead of cream sauces, butter, and gravies.
* Don't serve meat more than once a day; favor beans, fish, turkey, and chicken over red meats; buy lean meats.
* Don't serve more than three or four eggs per week; when baking, substitute two egg whites for every whole egg called for in the recipe, or use a no-cholesterol egg substitute.

✳

Guideline #4: Go Easy on the Sugar

Long before fat became our favorite dietary villain, refined sugar was the ingredient people feared (and craved) most. Nowadays, it's pretty difficult to avoid the stuff. Sugar doesn't just come in candy, cookies, and cakes anymore. It is generously added to nearly every packaged or processed food on the shelf, from peanut butter to salad dressing, soup, canned vegetables, pizza, and frozen entrees. And while our fat consumption has inched downward, our sugar consumption has soared. Researchers estimate that the average American child gets nearly twenty-five percent of total calories from sugar.

But the good news is that sugar is not as bad for people as was once believed. According to a Sugars Task Force convened by the U.S. Food and Drug Administration, its worst fault is that it promotes dental cavities. On the other hand, it's not something you should allow your child to consume at will. Aside from adding calories to the diet, refined sugar has no nutritional value: no vitamins, no minerals, no protein, no fiber. So if your child fills up on sugary foods, she's going to have trouble getting all of the nutrients her body needs.

---- ✳ ----

Easy Changes: Reducing Sugar

- Satisfy your child's sweet tooth by serving foods that are naturally sweet, such as fruit, for desserts and snacks.
- Read labels to uncover hidden sources of sugar, and

go easy on foods that list any of the following as the first or second ingredient: brown sugar, corn sweetener, corn syrup, high-fructose corn syrup, dextrose, fructose, glucose, lactose, maltose, sucrose, maple syrup, honey, molasses, or fruit juice concentrate.

- Limit consumption of soft drinks, juice, punch, juice cocktails, and other sugar-water concoctions;
- Top breakfast cereals with sliced fruit instead of sugar.
- Top pancakes and French toast with all-fruit jam or fresh fruit instead of maple syrup.

Guideline #5: Go Easy on the Salt and Sodium

It's no secret that most American adults eat far more salt and sodium than our bodies need. The same is true of children. In fact, according to one study, the average child eats five to ten times more sodium than necessary.

Consider this: The typical two-year-old needs only about 300 milligrams of sodium daily to ensure proper regulation of fluids and blood pressure. If he eats one ounce of American cheese he'll get 335 milligrams; if he eats one ounce of pretzels he'll get 515 milligrams; and if he has a bowl of canned spaghetti and meatballs he'll consume a whopping 1,140 milligrams.

The experts recommend that kids eat no more than 2,400 milligrams of sodium daily, but many feel that 1,800 milligrams (the equivalent of about one teaspoon of table salt) would be an even better cap on salt consumption. Why? Because some studies have shown that children who have a higher intake of salt also tend to have higher blood pressure than their peers. And children with higher blood pressure tend to become adults with hypertension, which is a major risk factor for heart disease and stroke. High-sodium diets may also be involved in osteoporosis and stomach cancer.

However, sodium seems to affect some people more than others, and there's still no way to tell who will or won't be sensitive to it. So don't become a fanatic about this. In the spirit of being safe rather than sorry, moderate the sodium in your child's diet. It's easier to not acquire a taste for salt in childhood than to unlearn the taste for it as an adult.

Easy Changes: Reducing Salt

- Serve fewer packaged, frozen, processed, canned, and fast foods.
- Resist the urge to add salt to your child's food before serving it.
- Don't put a salt shaker on the dinner table; offer an "herb shaker" instead.
- When buying prepared foods for toddlers, check the sodium content; if it's high, look for a lower-sodium substitute.
- When cooking, use herbs, spices, lemon juice, and sesame seeds for seasoning instead of salt.
- Limit the availability of salty snack foods such as chips and pretzels.
- Buy low-salt products whenever possible.
- Choose fresh or plain frozen vegetables over canned ones.
- Choose fresh fish, poultry, and meat over canned or processed ones.

Guideline #6: Keep Your Child Moving

This may not sound like a *dietary* guideline, but exercise is as important to good health as a balanced diet. It is included in the official Dietary Guidelines mainly to stress the importance of maintaining a healthy weight. Among adults, overweight is considered a major risk factor for high blood pressure, heart disease, stroke, diabetes, certain types of cancer, arthritis, breathing problems, and other illnesses.

Although children under six tend to need very little encouragement to be active, many working parents today have to plan ahead to make sure there's time for their children to enjoy outdoor physical activity. It's worth the effort to do this. In fact, concentrating on getting your child outdoors for at least an hour a day is a much more valuable use of your time than worrying about the fat, sugar, or sodium content of your child's food, or worrying about how to get rid of half the Halloween candy your kid just brought home.

Vigorous exercise is also considered a far better remedy for childhood weight concerns than a restricted diet, and it's one of the best methods for improving heart function and raising HDL cholesterol (the kind that's good for the body).

✳

Easy Changes: Encourage Exercise

- If bad weather keeps you in the house, turn on some music and dance with your child.
- Walk or bike places with your child, instead of always driving the car.

- Make walking the dog with your child a daily routine.
- Suggest physical activities such as playing catch, practicing soccer, or jumping rope when your child complains she's bored.
- Set an example by exercising regularly and talking about how good it makes you feel.
- Use stairs instead of elevators and escalators whenever possible.
- Limit TV and computer time to less than two hours a day.

The Final Guideline

There is one more Dietary Guideline, but it has to do with alcohol consumption. I've left it out because there is no question that children under age six should *not* be drinking alcohol of any kind.

What they should be doing is sampling the variety of foods for which our country is so famous, and learning to enjoy a full and active lifestyle.

✕ THREE

Beyond Nutrition: How Development Affects Eating

Knowing *what* your child should eat—and getting her to eat it—are two entirely different matters. That's because eating entails so much more than good nutrition. It also involves nonfood factors such as age, development, growth rate, environment, temperament, and taste buds. And your discipline style and eating habits carry enormous influence.

That's why this chapter is devoted to helping you solve the typical eating challenges presented at different stages of your child's development. In the first half, covering birth to age two, you'll learn lots of hands-on techniques that will help you get feeding off to a good start. But by the time you get to the section on ages two and up, you'll be reading a lot about positive discipline—and if your kids are anything like mine, you'll need every tip you find!

1 HOW INFANTS EAT

AGE FLAG: BIRTH TO 4 WEEKS

FIRST FEEDINGS

For many women, feeding is one of the easiest—and most enjoyable—parts of having a new baby. "The first time I put my son Geoffrey to my breast, he just latched right on and started sucking," says Mary Mitchell, a mother of three. "I remember thinking it seemed so natural—like that was exactly what breasts had been made for. Later on, when I introduced the bottle, he took to that right away, too."

But it isn't always that easy. For many new mothers, those first feedings bring more frustration than fulfillment. "I'll never forget how difficult it was at first to feed my daughter Rachel," says Louise Howsmon, a mother of two. "There were some complications right after her birth, so we started off under a lot of stress. Then every time I put her to my breast, she either couldn't latch on properly or she'd latch on, take a few sips, and then fall asleep. By the second or third day, I was so upset and frustrated that I began dreading the feedings. But the nurses at the hospital and the lactation consultant were supportive and encouraging, so I stuck with it, and by the fifth or sixth day, Rachel caught on."

When Problems Occur

If your first feedings are more like Louise and Rachel's than Mary and Geoffrey's, you may feel extremely discouraged. When you've just survived nine months of pregnancy and an exhausting delivery, having difficulty feeding your baby may seem like a hopeless mess. You may even feel like a failure. But rest assured, the situation isn't hopeless and you aren't a failure.

All babies are born with a sucking reflex. But they aren't born with the knowledge that if they suck on a nipple they'll receive milk, and that milk will make them feel better. (Please note: in the sections covering birth to age one, milk refers to either breast milk or formula.) That is the first lesson they must learn to survive, and like everything else, some infants learn it more quickly than others.

"If your baby isn't a 'natural,' all it means is that you'll have to be a little more patient and persistent in getting feedings off the ground," notes Dr. Kathy Merritt. Here are some strategies that will help:

1. Before you begin a feeding, get comfortable in a chair or on a bed. Have a drink of water, milk, or juice, and try to relax. Try to calm your baby, too. (Rock her, sing softly to her, or swaddle her firmly in a soft receiving blanket.) Be sympathetic to the fact that everything that's happening to your child is brand new to her (and probably to you, too).
2. Position your baby so that her head is close to your breast (even if you plan to bottle feed). The warmth and scent of your body and the comfort of your embrace will help to calm her.
3. Lightly stroke her cheek on the side closest to your body. You can use your finger, or the nipple of your breast, or the bottle. But be sure you touch only the cheek that's closest to you. If you stroke both

cheeks or the outside one, or if you squeeze the cheeks to force her mouth open, she won't know what to do next.

4. Keep gently brushing your baby's cheek until she turns her head toward your touch and opens her mouth. This is called the rooting reflex; it comes in all babies, and it lasts for the first three to four months of life. As soon as your baby begins rooting, lightly touch the nipple against her lips. Once she feels it, she will automatically open wider, latch on to the nipple, and start to suck.

If you're breast-feeding, you may have to guide her a bit, to make sure both your nipple and most of the areola get inside her mouth. If she only sucks on your nipple, she won't get the milk she needs (her sucking motion must compress the areola to cause a flow) and you'll end up with very sore nipples. Also, once your baby starts to suck, make sure her nose isn't buried in the more pendulous part of your breast: she needs a clear passageway to breathe!

If you are bottle feeding your baby, angle the bottle until the fluid fills up the nipple. Otherwise she may gulp down too much air with her meal, and later on experience gassiness and discomfort.

The Importance of Patience

It may take some time to get all of this coordinated. Don't let that worry you. The main goal of early feedings is to get both of you started on a pleasant habit. And the practice will pay off. By the time real hunger hits your baby's tummy (about four or five days after birth) she'll be an old pro at eating. "For now, the most critical thing is to help your baby feel loved and secure during feedings," says registered dietitian Felicia Busch.

If you don't see any improvements in your baby's appetite or ability to suck after a few attempts, don't blame yourself or waste your energy feeling like a failure. Get help from your pediatrician (or, if you're breast-feeding, a lactation consultant). "There may be a subtle glitch in your feeding technique, the food supply, or your baby's neurological development," notes pediatrician Dr. Barbara Kirschner. "A trained observer can pinpoint such problems and help you address them early on, before feeding your baby becomes something you (and he) dread."

FEEDING ON DEMAND

Once the two of you have figured out the basics, your next question will be, "*When* do I feed him?"

The answer is simple: feed your newborn whenever he's hungry, or when he cries to be fed. In the beginning, it may be every hour and a half, every three hours, or sometimes every two and sometimes every four. "Different babies have different patterns of hunger, and their need for food varies from day to day and meal to meal, especially during the first weeks of life," explains Dr. Harris Lilienfeld. The average newborn needs six to eight brief feedings a day, spaced about two to two-and-a-half hours apart; some demand more (as many as ten or twelve); others, less.

Feeding your baby when she indicates she's hungry is known as feeding "on demand." It wasn't always the popular approach. Parents used to be cautioned to keep their infants on a strict schedule of feedings every three or four hours, and to ignore the baby if he cried for food too soon. At one point, it was for medical reasons (some experts thought that irregular feedings caused intestinal infections, but it turned out that the real problem was unpasteurized milk); at another point, it was for discipline reasons (some experts thought that a strict feeding schedule kept a baby from becoming spoiled). "But there was no science behind those beliefs," notes Dorothy Sendelbach, M.D., F.A.A.P., an assistant clinical professor of pediatrics at the University of Texas Southwestern Medical Center at Dallas. "Today, making a hungry baby wait for food is considered somewhat cruel."

The current belief is that the more you cater to your newborn's natural hunger pattern and the sooner you comfort him when he's crying, the calmer and more well-adjusted he'll be. "When you feed your baby on demand, you help him build a sense of security and trust," notes Dr. Sendelbach. "He learns that when he needs something, there's someone right there to provide it."

When Difficulties Occur

If you have difficulty with feeding on demand, it may be because you're harboring too many notions about how babies should or shouldn't behave. You may be getting too much outdated advice from older relatives and friends. Or you may feel like life has gotten so out of control since your baby was born that you crave a more predictable routine. It's best to try to give up any preconceived notions you have right now and ignore any well-meaning advice about getting your newborn onto a schedule.

"You can't spoil your baby, no matter how often you pick her up and 'give in' to her demands for food or comfort," notes Dr. Sendelbach. "Nor can you change your baby's appetite or need for food. The best judge of what your baby needs to eat, and when, is your baby."

Instead of worrying about how often or how much your child is eating, you should:

1. *Pay attention to his hunger cues.* Depending on your child's temperament and level of hunger, he may squirm, fuss, or give an ear-piercing scream when he thinks it's time for a meal. If it's been less than two hours since your baby's last feeding and you aren't sure whether he's fussing for food or comfort, check to see if he needs a diaper change or try soothing him first, advises Dr. Ayoob. If that doesn't help, you can safely assume he needs more milk.

   After a while, you'll probably get to know your child's distinctive hunger cry. When babies are ready for food, they tend to be very persistent with their crying, and they don't quiet down until they get something to eat. It's a matter of basic survival.

   It's usually pretty clear when they're full, too. They disengage from the nipple and turn away, float into dreamland, or settle back and smile to themselves in drowsy satisfaction. The better you get at reading (and responding to) these signals, the more contentedly your baby will eat at each new feeding.

2. *Screen out distractions during feedings.* Try to make feeding times as quiet, calming, and relaxing as possible—for you and your child. If you're at home, turn on the answering machine, go to a quiet room, and put on some soft music, if you like. Just be sure you don't sit near a pile of dirty dishes or laundry, or a desk stacked with bills or reminders of deadlines at work or at home. And don't get into a heated debate with your spouse.

If you have other children underfoot, plan ahead to distract them. As Mary Mitchell notes, "It was easy to find a quiet place to nurse when I only had one child. But when my second baby was born, I had a nineteen-month-old who wanted my attention every time I sat down to nurse. I learned to plan ahead and find toys and videos to distract him while I was feeding the baby, so he could be in the same room but not bothering me. A lot of times, I'd end up with the baby on one side, nursing, and the toddler on the other, reading a book."

Other parents go even further. As one woman admits, "Every time I sat down to feed the baby, my four-year-old would want to crawl all over me, or she'd start crying and fussing to get my attention. There were days when I had to lock myself in my bedroom during feedings, just to get some peace and quiet."

3. *Let your infant eat in peace.* Once your baby is contentedly sucking, all you have to do is sit back and let him enjoy his meal. If you're breast-feeding, you'll need to switch breasts at some point (usually after about ten minutes on the first side); if you're bottle feeding, you may want to switch arms at the

halfway point to give your baby another view on the
world. And if you have the kind of child who likes
to burp (some do, some don't), you may want to try
for one before you switch sides. Other than those
few interruptions, there's nothing else you should
do.

Studies show that when parents try to help their
babies eat—by frequently checking the formula
level, changing the feeding position, wiping the
baby's chin, waking the baby up and pushing the
nipple in and out, for instance—the babies end up
eating less. So if your baby's sucking contentedly,
let him be.

4. *Attend to your own needs.* If you have the kind of
baby who wants to suckle at your breast or sip from
the bottle for hours at a time, it doesn't mean you
should always comply. As Dr. Sendelbach observes,
"Anytime you begin to feel that if someone put a
ring around your neck you'd become a human pacifier, it's time to set some limits."

Most normal, healthy babies can get sufficient
food from a twenty- or thirty-minute feeding. After
that, if they still want to suck (and you're not up to
a prolonged feeding), a pacifier may be helpful, or
you can try distracting them (with a walk, a toy, or
some music, for instance).

As Baby Grows

Even if initial feedings go smoothly, your baby will
probably lose some weight during his first week home
from the hospital, especially if he's being breast-fed.
This is perfectly normal. It is not a reflection of inade-

quate breast milk, too little formula, improper feedings, or a dislike of the food. It's just something that happens to most babies. "Some babies regain and surpass their birthweight within the first few days, while others take a little longer," notes Dr. Merritt. "But I like to see a baby regain her birthweight by around two weeks, and then show a steady climb upward."

According to the AAP, *if a baby fails to regain his birthweight by three weeks of age, or is still losing weight after the first ten days of life, medical intervention is essential.* These symptoms indicate a failure to thrive and must be immediately addressed by a pediatrician.

This is why it's extremely important to have your newborn's weight checked a week after birth, and regularly thereafter during the first year of life. Your baby's personal growth chart is, and will continue to be, the best tool for determining whether or not she's eating enough and growing properly.

"It's also important to call your pediatrician between checkups, if you ever have questions or concerns about your child's eating or weight," notes Corinne Montandon. "You will not be able to relax during feedings or resist forcing food if you are fearful that your child is not getting enough."

------------------------------ ✳ ------------------------------

Bowel Movements

Someday you'll look back and laugh at how much you and your partner talked about your baby's elimination pattern. But for now it's worth noticing, since it's an indication of how her body is working. Here's what you can expect:

With breast-fed babies:

• Bowel movements may seem incredibly frequent at first (some parents change as many as ten soiled diapers a day, though the average is five). As time goes by, you'll probably see fewer and fewer, but the overall number may remain high until breast-feeding is over;

• The stools may be mushy, seedy, and mustard-colored (though your child may still grunt and groan to push them out);

• The movements may be sudden and explosive at first, due to your baby's immature digestive system, and your baby may pass a lot of gas.

With formula-fed infants:

• The normal rate of frequency ranges from more than one movement a day, to one movement every two or three days;

• Stools are usually soft (if they're hard, they come out in marblelike pellets, or cause pain or bleeding, your baby may be constipated);

• They may be accompanied by gas.

Once solid food is introduced:

• Stools will become more like an adult's: thick, dark, and stinky;

• In younger babies, bowel movements may reflect the previous day's meal in color or texture; even if something your baby ate comes out whole in his stool, there's no need to worry. It's a normal result of his immature digestive system.

According to Dr. Merritt, the time to call a doctor is when bowel movements:
* Are watery, smelly, and occurring more than four times between two feedings;
* Show signs of blood or mucus;
* Are small and hard like marbles; or
* Suddenly change in frequency.

WHEN A FULL BABY FRETS

Even when feeding is going smoothly and a baby is being perfectly nourished, he may act hungry soon after a feeding has ended, or stop in the middle of a feeding to cry and fuss. Such behavior can be both puzzling and frustrating for a parent. You may even begin to resent your child: here you're doing everything you're supposed to—why isn't *he* satisfied?

One thing you can be sure of: he's not crying because he wants to make you angry. And if he's gaining weight, sleeping well, and seems otherwise content, he's probably not still hungry. "It's possible that your baby needs to have a bowel movement," says Dr. Sendelbach. "Or he may be mistaking the pain of gas or air in his stomach for hunger and looking for relief in milk."

Another possibility is that your baby is going through a period of colic, or irritable crying. Many newborns have an unexplained tendency to cry inconsolably at certain times of day (usually when their parents would like to relax and eat dinner).

"You can offer some comfort by trying to burp your baby, or letting him suck on a bottle of water (no more than one or two ounces daily), a pacifier, or your own (clean) finger," says Dr. Sendelbach. It may also help to lie the baby on her stomach, swaddle her firmly in a receiving blanket, take her for a walk, or go for a ride in the car. But if nothing works, you may just have to wait it out.

If the constant crying seems totally random and is beginning to push you over the edge, or you think your baby may be sick, call your pediatrician right away. It's better to get help than to try to endure something so overwhelming alone.

AGE FLAG: 1 TO 4 MONTHS

MOVING TOWARD A SCHEDULE

After a few weeks of demand feeding, your milk supply (if you're breast-feeding) will be well-established, your baby's digestive system will be more mature and able to handle greater amounts of milk, and your baby will be more attuned to the idea that milk relieves hunger pains. At this point, you will probably notice that your baby is not only drinking more, but following a more regular meal schedule and stretching the time intervals between feedings. With some babies, this happens quickly, and with little outside input. These kids just seem to know how to put themselves on a schedule. With others it takes a little guidance. "But even those who seem most reluctant to start a routine can, by about four to six weeks of age, be coaxed," says Dr. Merritt.

The first thing to do is figure out the average length of time your baby can go between feedings, and then stretch it a bit. For example, say your baby usually wants to eat every two hours. You know she had a meal at 2 P.M., but she wakes up from a nap and starts crying at 3:30 P.M. Instead of jumping right in with more milk, first try to distract her for a while. You could rock her or show her a rattle, take her for a walk, or give her a tour of the bedroom.

If she starts screaming inconsolably, don't keep delaying her. "When you know your baby is starving, there is no reason not to feed her," notes Dr. Merritt. She may need the earlier feeding because she didn't get enough at the previous meal, or because she's going through a growth spurt (a common occurrence at around three, six, and nine weeks of age). On the other hand, if she doesn't seem to mind your distractions, keep them up. If you're lucky, you'll be able to make it to 4 P.M. before she absolutely insists on being fed.

If you can only make it to 3:45 P.M., that's okay, too. The idea is to gradually lengthen the time between feedings, bit by bit, day by day.

What if it gets to be 4 or 4:30 P.M. (time for a feeding), and your baby is still sleeping? You could wake her up and try to feed her (a more regular schedule during the day sometimes helps reduce the number of feedings a baby requests at night). However, if she's not interested or keeps falling back asleep, you shouldn't force the issue. If she doesn't want it, she probably doesn't need it.

Eventually, you'll begin to notice that your baby isn't as enthusiastic as before when you offer the bottle every two hours. He may nip at the nipple halfheartedly, or spend more time studying your face than sipping his milk. That's a good sign that he's ready to start eating at two-and-a-half- or three-hour intervals.

Irregular Babies

If, despite your best efforts, you can't get your child on a regular schedule, don't despair—and don't respond with a show of force. As Dr. Merritt notes, "A rigid approach is rarely the answer with a baby." Besides, you're probably not doing anything wrong. You may just have a child with an "irregular" temperament.

Back in the 1950s, Stella Chess, M.D., and Alexander Thomas, M.D., psychiatrists at New York University Medical Center in New York City, began a study to explore their belief that babies are born with innate differences in how they behave and react to the world around them. Thanks to their (still ongoing) study, many experts now agree that all of us are born with an inherited physiological bias—or temperament—that affects not only how we feel, react to things, and learn, but how other people react to us.

As part of their study, Drs. Chess and Thomas identified nine distinct temperamental traits, many of which relate to eating habits:

1. Activity level (how physically active a person tends to be);
2. Regularity (how predictable a person is in eating, sleeping and other biological functions);
3. Approach/withdrawal (how a person usually responds to a new stimuli such as a new food, new feeder, or new place mat);

4. Adaptability (how long it takes to adjust to change, such as moving from breast to bottle or formula to cow's milk);
5. Sensory threshold (the degree of sensitivity to sounds, smells, flavors, textures, and visual or other stimuli);
6. Intensity (how forcefully a person voices his opinions and reacts to things);
7. Distractibility (how easy or difficult it is to distract a person once he's engaged in a task);
8. Persistence/attention span (how long a person can focus on something, even when there are other distractions);
9. Quality of mood (how positive or negative the person tends to be).

They also demonstrated that from birth, babies vary considerably within each of these categories. Some are highly regular, for instance, and will eat and have a bowel movement at about the same time every day. Others are highly irregular and will feel hungry or have bowel movements at unpredictable intervals.

What to Do

If you have an "irregular" baby, the best you can do is ease her toward a more predictable routine by trying to schedule feedings for about the same time every day, in the same place, even in the same chair. But never force your child to eat or leave him to cry inconsolably when he's hungry. "Otherwise, you may end up with a baby who doesn't eat at all," says Dr. Sendelbach. Instead, shoot for small improvements. And do not, under any circumstances, listen to advice from parents who had "regular" babies: they have no idea what you're going through!

If nothing seems to work, you may have to find ways simply to survive this period of your child's life. An irregular eating schedule won't harm your baby, and it doesn't foretell problems in your child's future. It just means you have to be a little more relaxed in your expectations about eating behaviors—and more creative in finding ways to get the rest and support *you* need.

✳

Spit-Up Strategies

Spitting up is one of the few things that aren't cute about a new baby. But nearly half of all babies do it (just look at the shoulder area of any new parent's shirt), and it's usually after a satisfying meal. Fortunately, the habit is harmless and tends to disappear once a baby starts sitting up or walking.

Why do babies spit up? In newborns, it's sometimes related to physical development, notes Dr. Sendelbach. "But commonly, it's a result of overfeeding or holding the baby in an awkward position." To minimize spit-ups:

* Never force your baby to finish a bottle or nurse for more than twenty minutes at a time;
* Try burping your child in the middle of a feeding instead of at the end;
* Feed your baby in a reclining—rather than flat—position;
* Put your baby upright (as in a stroller or front-pack) for a while immediately after meals;

- Elevate the head of your baby's crib mattress if she usually naps right after a meal;
- Avoid bouncing and jiggling your baby right after a meal.

CALL YOUR DOCTOR if:

- You notice any blood when your child spits up;
- He chokes and gags on the spit-up;
- Its color is brown or green instead of milky white; or
- It shoots straight across the floor (as in projectile vomiting).

MOVING FROM BREAST TO BOTTLE

Many women who breast-feed also want their babies to learn to drink from a bottle so they can return to work, get more rest, or enjoy an occasional evening out. Others are ready to switch from breast-feeding to bottle feeding by around the third month.

You can, of course, go directly from breast-feeding to cup feeding; however, if you plan to stop breast-feeding completely before your baby is six months old, you should switch to bottle feeding first unless your baby is a whiz with the cup. During most of this initial year of life, breast milk and formula supply the bulk of a baby's nutrients, and few infants under six months old are proficient enough at cup drinking to get all they need without a nipple. Even those who are may miss the comfort and pleasure that sucking provides.

Here are some additional hints:

- If you plan to continue breast-feeding, but want to offer an occasional (or supplemental) bottle, wait until your milk supply has been well-established and breast-feedings are going smoothly before you offer that first bottle. But don't wait too long. "The longer after two months you wait to introduce the bottle," says Dr. Schmitt, "the more strongly your infant will initially reject it." Once bottle feedings are accepted, he adds, you should offer at least three bottles a week.

- If you plan to give up breast-feeding entirely, give your baby time to get used to the bottle before making the final switch. Start with one bottle feeding a day, at the same meal every day. "Choose whatever meal is best for your baby and your schedule," advises Dr. Merritt. Then, wait until the first bottle is well accepted before adding another to the daily routine.

  This gradual approach will give your breasts time to slowly reduce their milk production, making painful engorgement less likely. If your breasts do become uncomfortably full when you aren't planning to feed, hand-express some milk to relieve the pressure without stimulating milk production.

- Use expressed breast milk for the first bottle feedings. The familiar taste may make acceptance of the new nipple easier. Once the artificial nipple is accepted, introduce formula.

- Have your spouse or another caregiver be the one to introduce the bottle and, if possible, take over the bottle feedings. If your baby sees you or smells your breast milk, he's not going to be easily tempted by a bottle of formula.

- Present the bottle when your child is hungry but not famished. Otherwise, complete rejection is likely.

• If your child resists the bottle at first (most breast-fed babies do), you can either offer your breast and try again tomorrow or present an ultimatum: bottle or nothing for that meal. "The first is the kinder approach, but it may also take more time for the bottle to be accepted," notes Dr. Merritt. "The second will work within a day or two, but it will also involve a lot more crying." Choose the strategy with which *you* feel most comfortable.

NIGHTTIME FEEDINGS

In the earliest weeks of life, most babies require two or three feedings during the night to satisfy their nutritional needs. Physically, they aren't able to consume all the calories they require to sustain their growth during daytime meals. Even the best of eaters under a month old usually can't last for more than five hours between feedings at night.

Fortunately, as babies gain more weight and consume more milk during the day, they begin to decrease their demands for crib-side service after the sun has set. But there's no telling when that magic moment of sleeping through the night will come. A (very lucky) friend of mine tells me that both of her daughters slept through the night from the day they came home from the hospital. My first son was sleeping through his night feedings by six weeks, but my second son didn't reach that milestone for months.

Even if every other new baby you know who's your child's age can go the distance at night and yours can't, don't panic. It won't help to feel angry at your child or yourself. Nor should you try to ignore your baby's cries to "teach her a lesson."

The bottom line is that if a baby under four months old feels hungry at night, it's not her fault. She simply needs more time to grow and mature until her body is able to take in all the food it needs during the day. Understanding this can help you feel more patient and sympathetic when the sleepless nights seem to go on and on.

If they're wearing you out, ask your partner to take on the night feeding or hire an overnight babysitter so you can get more rest. That will do far greater good than trying to force your hungry baby to sleep.

2 HOW BABIES EAT

AGE FLAG: 4 TO 6 MONTHS

THE TURNING POINT

By the time your cherub is five or six months old, it will be far less likely that nutrition is the issue in any remaining nighttime wakings. By this age, late-night nips are usually a matter of habit: your baby has come to enjoy seeing you and having a quiet snack when the rest of the world is asleep. This is a very different matter from hunger, and you can take steps to discourage it (if you're desperate to reclaim your right to a good night's sleep). Some or all of the following strategies may help:

1. Schedule what you hope will be the final feeding of

the night for right before your own bedtime. If your
baby's asleep by then, wake him up to feed him. If
he's too sleepy to get a full tummy of milk, don't
try to force the feeding. Let him drink what he can.
With some babies, this last-minute snack can make
the difference between a middle-of-the-night feeding and an early morning breakfast.

2. To reduce the frequency of night feedings (from two
   or three to one, for instance) offer more food at the
   one time you're most willing to keep, and less at the
   others.

3. Always put your baby to bed—in the day and the
   night—when she's drowsy but still awake. In other
   words, don't let her fall asleep in the middle of the
   feeding and then gently place her in her crib. If
   she's accustomed to drifting off with a nipple in her
   mouth, that's the first thing she'll think of when she
   awakens at night. (All babies experience partial
   awakenings as they move from one phase of the
   sleep cycle to another.) If you can get your baby in
   the habit of falling asleep on her own, she'll be less
   likely to cry out for food during her partial awakenings, and more likely just to put herself back to
   sleep.

4. If you're the type who can tough it out when your
   baby cries, try delaying your response time by five
   or ten minutes when you first hear him whimpering
   for a nocturnal snack, says Dr. Merritt. Once he realizes you aren't going to jump right up and serve a
   meal, he may give up and go back to sleep on his
   own. If he doesn't, go to him, but don't pick him up
   right away. Instead, keep the light off and try to
   calm him down by rubbing his back or turning on a

lullaby tape or musical toy. (If you're breast-feeding, it will definitely help if another caregiver responds to these nighttime wakings. When a baby can see or smell his milk supplier, he isn't easily distracted.)

If your baby can't be calmed in his crib, pick him up and try rocking or walking with him. Eventually, if he doesn't go back to sleep, you may have to give in and feed him. "If so, make it a brief, nonemotional feeding," advises Dr. Merritt. (You don't want him to think this is a time to snuggle, or play and have fun; you can always encourage those pleasures during daylight hours.) And don't feel that you've failed if you end up feeding. If nothing else, you've taken a step toward lengthening the interval between late-night meals. There's always tomorrow night. . . .

5. If you're bottle feeding at night, gradually reduce the amount of formula you offer (with your pediatrician's okay). Or slowly dilute the nighttime servings with water, until after a few days there's only water in the bottle. Many babies will figure it isn't worth the effort to wake up for just water.

   If you're breast-feeding, gradually reduce the amount of time you nurse at night. Even if this doesn't cure night wakings right away, it will help shift your baby's calorie intake to daytime feedings, making it easier and easier for her to give up moonlight meals.

6. If you haven't already done so, try moving your baby out of your room into his own. The longer distance from his bed to yours may make it easier for both of you to give up the nighttime rendezvous.

As you employ any of these techniques, keep in mind that even if your child gets over needing a nighttime feeding, she may still awaken and cry at night. At that point you're dealing with a sleep issue, not an eating issue. (For tips on solving sleep-related problems, see *Sleep: How to Teach Your Child to Sleep Like a Baby*, another book in the *Child* Magazine parenting series.)

WEANING WITH GRACE

Learning to use a cup and a spoon can be either exciting or frustrating for your baby, depending on when and how you approach them. If you start weaning too soon, because other people tell you your baby *ought* to be doing this or that, the result is more likely to be frustration. "If you wait too long, however, and your baby becomes overly attached to her bottle or breast-feedings, you may end up facing some surprisingly firm resistance," notes Dr. Kirschner.

"By about six months, most babies are no longer quite as content as they used to be in the role of backseat driver," adds Felicia Busch. "They're more aware of the world around them, and more eager to get involved in the decisions that affect them."

The solution is to watch for clues that your baby is ready, and then proceed at the pace she dictates.

INTRODUCING THE CUP

Whether you plan to move from breast to cup or from bottle to cup, a good time to start preparing for this

transition is when your baby is six months old if you're
breast-feeding; four to six months old if bottle feeding.

The sooner you start, however, the less likely it is
that you'll see immediate results. According to Dr.
Schmitt, most babies aren't able to pick up a cup and
drink freely from it until they're between nine and
eighteen months old. On the other hand, if you wait too
long to introduce the cup, you may encounter a stubborn child who would rather stage a hunger strike than
give up her precious bottle (or breast). Younger babies
tend to be more easily convinced than older ones to
change established routines.

"At whatever point you begin, be sure to start
slowly," notes Montandon. It will also help if you:

- *Use a durable plastic cup with a spill-proof lid.* You
  can find such cups everywhere these days: in baby
  catalogs, retail outlets, and even grocery stores. And
  there's no shortage of colors, sizes, and styles, so if
  your baby rejects one type of cup, you can easily find
  another to try.
- *Make sure your child is comfortably seated.* You can
  put him in his high chair, his stroller, an infant seat,
  or your lap. It doesn't matter. Where he sits isn't as
  important as making sure he is firmly supported in
  an upright position.
- *Make sure your baby isn't starving.* If he's at the
  point where all he cares about is getting food into his
  tummy, it's not a good time to introduce a new eating
  appliance. Choose the meal when he tends to be most
  compliant, and wait until he's had a chance to take
  the edge off his hunger before you offer the cup.
- *Experiment with different fluids.* If you have the type

of baby who balks at most changes in routine, start out with whatever food she usually drinks: breast milk (expressed) or formula. The familiar taste may make the new container seem less threatening. On the other hand, some babies will resist if their favorite food is offered in a new way. Try putting water or watered-down juice in the cup (and don't offer those drinks in the bottle).

• *Expect very little at first.* Whatever you use, start out small, both in the amount of fluid you put in the cup and in your expectations of how much your child will drink. Hold the cup to his lips and let a tiny bit of fluid slip into his mouth. Then withdraw the cup and give him a chance to taste and swallow. Don't be concerned if much of the liquid dribbles down his chin at first. "It doesn't necessarily mean he doesn't like it," notes Dr. Merritt. "It just means he needs more practice to perfect his technique."

If, after the first sip, he seems interested in another, oblige him; if he cries, turns away, gags, or knocks the cup out of your hand, just call it a day. There's no Olympics for cup drinkers, so why shoot for early achievement?

• *Persist, but don't insist.* If your child continues to resist cup drinking, just put the cup (either empty or with a small amount of fluid in it) on his high-chair tray during meals. That way he can get comfortable with the new device without feeling pressured to use it. If he's the kind of kid who likes to do things on his own, he may surprise you some day and try to drink from it. If he doesn't, suggest a sip now and then, but don't insist.

• *Gradually add more fluid.* As your child begins to

accept the cup, add more and more liquid, until she's drinking as much from the cup as she normally would from a bottle at that meal (this may take a few months). Then eliminate that bottle (or breast-feeding) and work on switching from nipple to cup at another meal. The idea is to divide and conquer, meal by meal.

INTRODUCING THE SPOON

Feeding a baby her first spoonful of food is an event many new parents anticipate with eager excitement. There are lots of reasons why. One is that it's something new, to break the routine of milk feedings. Another is that it signals growth and development on the part of the child, and makes a parent feel a certain sense of accomplishment ("Wow! We got her to survive on milk, now let's try some *real* food!"). In addition, spoon feeding seems more normal to us. *We* don't survive on liquids alone, so how can a baby?

Along with the excitement, however, comes a lot of unrealistic expectations. "For example," notes Dr. Sendelbach, "many parents think that the sooner they feed their baby cereal, the sooner he'll sleep through the night. But the research shows that isn't the case. Adding cereal to the bottle, or feeding it on a spoon *does not* improve nighttime sleeping."

Another common misconception is that the baby will love solid food right away. The fantasy is that your cute little baby, bedecked in a cute little bib, will swallow her first taste of cereal, pause to smile gratefully at you, and then open wide for more. Most parents even imagine themselves dressed in clean clothes for this event, with a confident smile on their face as they scoop out mush from the bowl.

All too often, reality looks more like this: You put your clean, bibbed baby in the high chair. You trick her into opening her mouth for the spoon. You quickly deposit the food on her tongue, and then sit back to enjoy her reaction. She shoots you a look of surprise and horror, and then cries desolately as it dribbles down her chin.

Improving the Odds

The key to avoiding frustration is to approach spoon feeding as a process rather than an event. Chapter Two outlines the physical and nutritional issues surrounding the introduction of solid foods (see page 47). Here are some additional tips for success with the spoon:

- *Let your baby watch you eat.* That will whet both his appetite and his curiosity about nonliquid foods. "A lot of times, you can tell a child is ready to try out a spoon because he's so intent when watching other people eat," notes Dr. Merritt. "He may even lean across his high-chair tray and put his hand out toward your plate." That's a clear sign of readiness.

- *Sit him in a high chair.* Your baby must be sitting up for spoon feedings, for safer swallowing, so make sure you have proper seating arrangements. If you try to use your lap, you'll have a tough time supporting him while juggling the spoon and the bowl. A better choice is a high chair or booster seat with a tray. That way you can sit comfortably, keep the food out of his reach, and face him as you feed him.

- *Work around your baby's schedule.* Plan the first spoon feedings for a time of day when your baby is usually happy, alert, and open to new experiences. Many babies, for instance, are so hungry at breakfast or so tired and cranky at supper that they don't take kindly to changes in routine.

  Also, time your introduction of solid food for when your child is hungry but not famished. Let him suck on the bottle or breast-feed for a while first, to take the edge off his hunger. But don't let him get so full of milk that he won't be interested in trying a new type of food. You can always offer more milk after the spoon feeding is done.

- *Use a spoon with a long handle and small bowl* (a baby spoon, a demitasse spoon, or an iced-tea spoon), to make feedings easier for both of you. Short-handled baby spoons are better for when your child can feed herself.

- *Prepare for a mess.* Cover the floor with a splat mat, shower curtain liner, absorbent towel, or newspapers; cover the baby with a good bib; and cover yourself with a towel or apron, to protect your clothes from globs of goo. Keep some paper towels within reach. "Feeding a baby can be a very messy affair," notes Corinne Montandon, "but you're less likely to mind if you expect and prepare for it."

- *Introduce the food first.* Before you give your baby his first mouthful, put a little dollop of whatever you're serving on his tray, so he can touch and explore it a bit. Then put a dab of the food on the spoon and slip the edge into your baby's mouth. He'll probably suck it off (although he may spit it out). If he opens wider, push the spoon a little farther back, to the middle of his tongue, to make swallowing more likely. But don't be discouraged if the food you just deposited comes sliding back out as soon as you remove the spoon. If your baby is developmentally ready for spoon feedings, he'll soon start swallowing more than he spits out. (If he keeps on spitting food out, he's probably not ready for this; wait a couple of weeks and try again.)

- *Watch for clues that your baby has had enough.* She may turn her head away from you, start spitting the food out, refuse to open her mouth, start acting fussy, or push your hand or the food away. Don't try to get her to change her mind by making choo-choo noises or trying other tricks. In addition to teaching her about food, you're teaching her to recognize and follow her own internal cues about hunger and appetite. And you're showing her that her opinions are wanted and respected.

When to Worry

Anytime you don't feel spoon feeding is progressing as you expected, check with your pediatrician. There may be some minor changes in what or how you're feeding your child that will help. "This is especially important if your child is seven or eight months old and refusing to accept solids," adds Dr. Sendelbach. "At that point, if he's still hooked on the bottle, he may begin developing an aversion to nonliquid textures and tastes, and his nutrition may be compromised."

AGE FLAG: 6 TO 12 MONTHS

PERFECTING NEW SKILLS

Once your baby has been formally introduced to the cup and the spoon, his next challenge will be learning to use them. He'll need time to hone his skill at swallowing solids before he can move on to munching and crunching.

But learning to eat won't be the only thing on your baby's mind. He'll be trying to master a lot of other mechanics over these next few months, such as sitting, crawling, standing, and walking, not to mention reaching, grasping, and moving objects from one place to another. "As all of these complicated skills develop, his urge for independence will continue to grow, and there'll be lots more opportunities for the two of you to butt heads," adds Felicia Busch. He'll be touching things you don't want him to, refusing foods you want him to eat, knocking things off his high chair, and crying for attention when you're trying to cook. During feedings, he may even grab the spoon from your hand and insist that he feed himself (even though he clearly can't).

Be prepared to face whatever balky or resistant behavior your baby dishes out with patience and love. "Try to think of his attempts to gain the upper hand as a good sign," notes psychotherapist James Windell. "He's not trying to be difficult; he's trying to learn and grow and explore the world he lives in." When he asserts himself, it means not only that all these developmental milestones are proceeding normally, but that your baby has grown confident enough in your love to try and defy you now and then.

Ensuring Smooth Sailing

With feeding, your most important goal right now should be to "help your baby feel like eating is something he *wants* to do, rather than something you're making him do," stresses Felicia Busch. Here's how to keep that message clear:

- *Let your baby get involved.* One good strategy is to place a spoon within her reach as you feed her. It may be another nine or so months before your child can comfortably feed herself with a spoon, but for now she can at least practice picking it up, holding it, waving it around, aiming it toward her bowl, and lapping up whatever sticks to it with her tongue.
- *Keep your expectations low.* There are no hard-and-fast rules for what a baby should eat, how much she should eat at any given meal, when she should eat particular foods, what combinations of foods should be eaten together, or how long mealtimes should last. If you find yourself getting angry or frustrated because your baby is refusing foods, playing with her food, or making too much of a mess, take a break. Walk away, take a few deep breaths, and remind yourself that her behavior is not only normal, it will not last forever. She will outgrow this stage and eventually eat more like a civilized human being.
- *Make all foods seem equal.* In other words, don't force your baby to eat her peas before she can have her pudding. Instead, offer a little of this and a little of that throughout the meal.
- *Add texture gradually.* Once your child becomes comfortable with pureed, strained, and mashed foods, introduce more texture to her diet: cottage cheese with lumps, for instance, or bits of scraped apple, coarsely pureed vegetables, or finely ground meat. This will

help broaden her food horizons and prepare her to
eventually bite and chew.

INTRODUCING FINGER FOODS

Sometime between seven and eight months of age,
your baby will become accomplished enough at grab-
bing and guiding to begin making more-solid foods
(soft crackers, cubes of whole-wheat bread, and
cooked vegetables, for instance) a serious part of her
daily menu. At around nine to twelve months, she'll
develop a pretty good pincer grip and be ready to feed
herself tiny foods such as peas and raisins. "Always
try to encourage her abilities and interests in the self-
feeding arena," stresses Corinne Montandon. Independence at the dinner table is the inevitable next step in
eating development; in addition, finger foods will feed
her hunger for control, as well as her body.

The most important consideration when offering
finger foods is: Could my baby choke on this? "Even
kids who have sprouted teeth by now should not be
considered accomplished chewers," notes Corinne
Montandon. "So be sure to avoid hard foods like raw
carrots and pears, chunks of meat or poultry, hot
dogs, peanuts, and popcorn." Opt for soft foods with a
melt-in-the-mouth quality, such as no-salt rice cakes,
low-sugar cereals, chunks of ripe, soft fruit (such as
banana, peach, cantaloupe, or mango), and cubes of
soft cheese.

Also, consider the nutritional quality of what you are
serving, especially at snack time. At this early age, kids
aren't going to be begging for cookies and chips, or
even white bread and sugary cereals—unless you get

them into the habit. "Their taste preferences are completely open to suggestion right now, so if you steer them toward healthy foods, they're more likely to grow up wanting and enjoying them," notes Hess.

Start Small

When you present the finger-food portion of your baby's meal, don't overdo it. Place three or four pieces of food directly on her tray or on a nonbreakable plate, and let her start sampling at her own pace; after she's eaten about half her initial supply, replace the missing pieces. If her plate is too full, she may be tempted to grab everything and stuff it into her mouth; or she may feel so overwhelmed that she'll just dump it all onto the floor. If you add a little at a time, she'll be more likely to want to touch and taste what's on her plate.

If your baby just wants to play with her finger foods, let her (within reason, of course; you needn't allow her to decorate the rug with it). "At this age, children are very tactile—they love to touch and squish and mush and mash anything they can get their tiny hands on," says Corinne Montandon. "Sometimes, playing with a new food helps build their bravery for trying it."

As your child's acceptance of finger foods grows, increase the portions; eventually, they should overtake the mushier parts of her meal.

Things a Baby Shouldn't Eat

As your baby's ability to consume finger foods grows, so will her interest in sampling other items such as dirt, dust balls, bits of old food left on the floor, coins, pills, plants, and small toy parts. He has no way of knowing just yet what is and isn't edible, so it's your job to keep his fast little fingers away from harmful nonfoods.

"It is especially important to keep alcohol, medicine, and poisonous household products out of sight and out of reach," notes Ann A. Hertzler, Ph.D., R.D., C.H.E., a professor and Extension specialist with the Virginia Cooperative Extension, at Virginia Tech in Blacksburg, Virginia. "Don't take any chances," she adds. "Thousands of children ingest poisonous substances in their own homes each year." Just because your baby doesn't seem interested in the box of detergent under your sink today, it doesn't mean that tomorrow, when you turn your head for half a second, he won't manage to reach it, grab it, and lick the powder off the top. Babies can be amazingly quick when getting into mischief.

REDUCING MILK FEEDINGS

By the time your baby is about nine months old, he should be getting enough nutrients from solid foods to survive with fewer breast-milk and/or formula feedings. Now's the time to start preparing for the day when you'll wean your baby completely from the breast or bottle. That's not to say you should do it right away, but you should prepare for it. Here's how:

- Once your baby is eating three solid meals a day, with two or three finger-food snacks, offer the bottle or breast no more than three or four times a day with meals. (You can save the fourth feeding for just before bedtime.) If your child requests more frequent bottles or breast-feedings, find alternative ways to comfort her, such as holding her, distracting her with a toy, going for a walk, or offering a cup of water.

- If you tend to nurse your child every time you hold him, or use the bottle or breast in times of distress, break those habits now. They teach your child to associate food with comfort rather than with hunger. And they practically guarantee a prolonged attachment to breast or bottle. Don't hug and comfort your child less; just avoid using food when a kiss, a Band-Aid, a quick cuddle, or a lullaby would work as well.
- If your child has a strong need to suck even when he's not actually hungry, encourage him to use a pacifier or suck on his thumb instead of turning to the breast or bottle. Again, he needs to learn the difference between feeling hungry and wanting comfort.
- If you haven't already done so, introduce the cup. Don't wait until you're ready to switch completely to cup feedings, or you may encounter a great deal of unnecessary resistance. It's far better to let your child practice cup-drinking skills when he doesn't feel an immediate threat to his usual mode of drinking.
- When you offer feedings, insist that your child take them sitting down. As his desire and ability to move around and explore increases, he'll become more impatient with these sit-down meals and will eventually decide that sticking with the bottle isn't worth it; he'd rather get up and go. He'll have no incentive to make that decision, however, if you regularly allow him to carry his beloved bottle around and sip from it at his leisure.
- Never put your baby to bed with his bottle. This not only presents a greater risk of tooth decay and ear infections, it can lead to a dependency on bottles to

get to sleep. Similarly, do not allow your baby to fall asleep at your breast. You can't always prevent this, of course, but whenever possible, put her into her crib when she's drowsy but not asleep.

All of these steps will help reinforce the idea that "breasts and bottles are for nutrition, not comfort," notes Dr. Merritt. "That, in turn, will make it easier when it comes to weaning your baby completely from the breast or bottle."

3 HOW TODDLERS EAT

AGE FLAG: 1 TO 2 YEARS

ALMOST EATING LIKE YOU

By the time you celebrate your child's first birthday, she'll probably be eating her meals at the table like the rest of the family. And almost anything you serve will be suitable for her. That's not to say she'll always eat what you offer or prefer the foods you do. But she will be physically capable of eating what everyone else is.

"However, you'll need to make a few modifications so she can easily feed herself," says Corinne Montandon. Kids this age are more likely to eat eagerly if:

- Their food is properly cut and easy to chew and swallow;
- You provide a kid-size spoon, with a short handle;
- You put their finger foods directly onto their (clean) high-chair tray, rather than onto a slippery plate;

- Their bowl is sturdy, steady, and nonbreakable (the best choice is one with a suction mechanism at the bottom to prevent it from sliding across the tray);
- Their cup is nonbreakable and has some sort of spill-proof lid;
- You don't offer too many different foods at once;
- You don't offer too much of any one food (it's always better to offer seconds);
- You don't fill your child up on juice and junk foods right before scheduled meals;
- You let your child eat more when he's unusually hungry, and less when he's not.

Food Resistance

In addition to eating more like an adult, your child will be acting less like a baby. Her growth rate will slow, and she'll be far more active than you ever dreamed possible a year ago; plus, her motor skills will probably amaze you. Her new mobility may make mealtimes a bit more difficult (since she can now run away when you say it's time to eat, and her aim when pitching carrots will be much improved); also, she may become so involved in doing and exploring that she forgets she needs food.

(We'll talk a lot more about how to cope with oppositional table behaviors in the next two sections, covering ages two to six. If you need help in this area before your child is two, don't worry. You're not alone. Most kids enter the stage known as the "terrible twos" months before they actually turn two—so feel free to read ahead.)

On the positive side, one-year-olds tend to be fairly

agreeable (compared to two-year-olds) and open to new experiences, so this is a good time to expose your child to new foods. Variety on the table not only translates to better nutrition, it cultivates an early appreciation for different tastes, textures, and types of food.

If you're lucky, your baby will revel in the gastronomic delight of this new stage of eating. You may even be alarmed, sometimes, at the size of her appetite. As Carol Spelman, a mother of two, observes, "My one-year-old, Julia, has yet to refuse anything I've put in front of her. In fact, sometimes I wonder whether I'm overfeeding her because it seems that she would eat all day if I let her. But I enjoy feeding her because she eats with such enthusiasm, and I know from experience with my first child that those days are short-lived."

Not all one-year-olds eat with such gusto, of course. And you shouldn't feel discouraged if you have the kind of baby who routinely rejects whatever you offer. This is also an age when food preferences become more pronounced, and some children become more suspicious of anything new. In the chapter on picky eaters, you'll find some great tips for building your child's taste bud bravery. But for now, what you need to know is that most healthy children this age—including those who seem to be overeating, and those who seem to be undereating—are consuming the perfect amount of food for their individual bodies.

COMPLETING THE WEANING PROCESS

If you haven't already weaned your baby from breast or bottle, now's the time to think seriously about when and how to do it. Your child is in a new nutritional and developmental stage, and it's far more important now than it was six months ago for her to switch her allegiance from lap feedings to table feedings, and from nipple to cup and spoon. Here are some issues and tips you should consider as you prepare for the final weaning.

Ending Bottle Feedings

For bottle-fed babies, the twelve-month mark is considered a good time to bite the bullet. Kids this age are usually physically capable of drinking all the liquids they need from a spill-proof cup. And most have reached a stage when they would rather get eating done quickly so they can rush off to enjoy the world than sit and suck on a bottle in someone's lap.

Of course, many one-year-olds cling to their bottle feedings, and many parents don't mind if their child seeks comfort from the bottle well into their toddler and preschool years. "I'm not rigid about telling parents they have to get their child off the bottle by a certain age," says Dr. Merritt. "In some households, the only way to get the rest of the family dressed and out the door for school and work is to let the toddler sip on her bottle. You have to look at what works in your life, as well as in your baby's.

"But you should also keep in mind that the older your baby gets, the more attached she'll become to her bottle, and the harder it'll be to take it away," adds Dr. Merritt.

Also, if you allow your child to use her bottle as a security blanket (and sip from it all day long), it may interfere with her appetite and her ability to broaden her social and educational horizons.

Move Slowly

This doesn't mean you should go cold turkey with bottle weaning as soon as you bake your baby's first birthday cake. Instead, gradually move through the following steps:

1. Begin working toward total weaning when nothing special is happening in your household, and you aren't under any unusual stress. Do not attempt it if your family is moving, your baby is getting a new caregiver, your baby or someone else in the house is ill, or there's been a recent death or other turmoil in your lives. During such times, a baby needs a dependable source of comfort, just as adults do.

2. Before you give each regularly scheduled bottle, offer your child cow's milk in a cup first, to get him used to a new way of drinking. (He may surprise you and quickly prefer it!) If he resists, offer his usual formula in the cup to get him going.

3. Once your child is confident with the cup, eliminate the bottle completely from one of his regular daily feedings, and offer only the cup. Make sure you pick a meal at which your baby usually has a good appetite but is not deliriously hungry (as many kids are just after waking up, for instance).

4. After three or four days, or once your child has adjusted to the disappearance of the first bottle, eliminate another from a regularly scheduled meal.

5. Repeat step four until all bottles have been elimi-

nated, making sure you give your child enough time to adjust at each stage.

Getting rid of the very last bottle is sometimes easy, because by then the child has lost interest in bottle feeding. But some children hold on for dear life. With them, you need to be creative.

Dr. Sendelbach says that she was able to convince one of her children to give up his last bottle by taking off the nipple and putting in a straw. "Our son was happy, because he still had his bottle," she says, "and we were happy because he wasn't sucking on a nipple. Eventually, when the novelty wore off, he stopped asking for the bottle."

Other parents have developed special rituals for getting rid of the last bottle. "When a cousin of mine was about four, she used to love going to the beach," recalls Dr. Merritt. "So her parents finally convinced her to give up her bottles by having her 'throw them to the fishies' during a visit to the beach."

If all else fails, go ahead and use the cold turkey approach and just throw the bottles away. "If you know that you're not the kind of person who can refuse your child his bottle when he starts crying or begging for it, then a fast ending may be the best solution," notes Dr. Merritt. "It will not cause your child any undue or lasting trauma if you just get rid of the bottles and tell your child, 'I'm sorry, honey. The bottles are gone.' "

6. If after all the bottle feedings have ended, your toddler still asks or cries for a bottle now and then, hold her in your lap and comfort her, advises Dr. Merritt. If she's thirsty, offer a drink in the cup. But don't

go back to bottle feeding, or you'll have to start the weaning process all over again.

Ending Breast Feedings

Deciding when to stop breast-feeding is a very personal decision that has as much to do with your baby's needs as your own. "There is no right or wrong time to stop," notes Dr. Merritt. "Some women nurse their babies for as little as a week or two; some nurse for six or more months, and a few continue to breast-feed well into their child's second or third year—or beyond."

Many children decide on their own when they're done with breast-feeding. My first son lost interest at six months, when he discovered he enjoyed solid food as much as breast milk; my second son's interest tapered off around the nine-month mark, just before he started walking. In both cases, I wasn't dying to give up our special feedings, but my babies were, so I decided to follow their lead and found other ways to maintain our intimacy.

You'll know your baby is ready for weaning if he:

- Repeatedly refuses the breast, or wriggles and squirms when you hold him in the usual breast-feeding position;
- Tends to nurse intensely for a few minutes, but then pulls away and acts fussy (even though he's not sick, already full, or teething);
- Bites you while nursing; or
- Becomes easily distracted during feedings.

If your child starts asking for more frequent feedings or resumes night feedings, lack of nourishment may be the problem—and weaning the solution.

Then, of course, there are those babies who never falter in their passion for the breast. Although you should wean a baby who indicates he's ready to stop, there's nothing wrong with continuing breast-feedings with a child who doesn't seem ready—as long as she's happy and healthy, you don't mind nursing her, and it's not interfering with her intake of solid foods. But be aware that after twelve months, children rarely initiate weaning on their own. So eventually, you'll have to be the one to close up the milk bar.

At whatever point you feel that you and/or your baby are ready for the final weaning, follow the steps outlined in the section on Ending Bottle Feedings (reread "Move Slowly," page 118, and substitute the words *breast-feeding* and *breast milk* wherever you see *bottle feedings* and *formula*).

4 HOW PRESCHOOL KIDS EAT

AGE FLAG: 2 TO 3 YEARS

THE AGE OF UNREASON

Not all two-year-olds are difficult, and not all parents feel like they're on the edge of losing their sanity when their children are in the "terrible twos." But a great many kids are, and an even greater number of parents do. So be prepared: this is the age when your fears about nutrition will likely give way to worries about eating behaviors.

Two-year-olds can be wonderful creatures. They're cute, capable, and charming; they speak in adorable and imaginative ways; they're curious and friendly; they love to play; and they're quite delicious when they run over and jump into your arms for a big, fat hug.

But that's only one side of being two. There are other, less-adorable habits that many perfectly normal two-year-olds display—such as screaming, hitting, biting, and throwing terrible temper tantrums to get their way. In the eating arena, they're notorious for annoying and defiant behaviors such as:

- Asking for one thing (like a peanut butter sandwich) and then, when you give it to them, demanding another ("I want turkey!");
- Refusing to eat anything at all;
- Eating only one food or one type of food for days on end, and then one day crying because you served it to them and they "hate" it;
- Crying because you did (or didn't) cut their food the right way, or you cut (or didn't cut) the crusts off their bread;
- Throwing a tantrum because they only want dessert, not lunch;
- Eating two bites of food and then wriggling out of their chair to go play;
- Screaming because you asked them to stop playing and eat;
- Refusing to eat at dinner, and then begging for food as soon as you've finished cleaning the kitchen;
- Throwing food they don't like onto the floor;
- Using their spoon as a drumstick on the table or on their bowl;
- Spilling drinks;

- Insisting that you stop trying to help them, and then wailing when they can't pick up the food themselves;
- Complaining because you served the food in the wrong way or in the wrong order—even if you're just following the routine your child has been insisting on all week.

It's important to convince yourself that all of these behaviors are perfectly normal for this age. Though they can be extremely frustrating, they are *not* worth fighting about.

THE TWO-YEAR-OLD'S AGENDA

Two-year-olds are not defiant and difficult on purpose, or just to bug their parents. They're on a developmental mission that's vital to their mental and emotional health. They've spent a lot of energy up to this point mastering complex physical skills such as sitting, crawling, walking, reaching, and grasping (not to mention drinking from a cup and eating from a spoon). Now they're ready to test their ability to master their universe. But at the same time, they desperately need to know that you're still there to love and care for them, just in case their plans crumble. These opposing inner struggles are what give two-year-olds the reputation of being "terrible."

"It's fairly typical for toddlers to not know what they want," says James Windell. "And though most of them are in love with saying the word *no,* they don't particularly enjoy hearing it."

Some children are only mildly rebellious at two and will only defy you in one or two areas; others will happily turn every request you make into an excuse not to cooperate. With all two-year-olds, however, eating can quickly become a favored battleground, since it involves all the necessary elements:

1. An issue that affects health and well-being;
2. A parent with definite ideas (about when, what, and how much food should be eaten);
3. A child with definite ideas (about when, what, and how much food should be eaten);
4. Regularly scheduled gatherings, where the two of you can disagree; and, most important,
5. A subject on which the child always gets the final say (after all, they're the ones with ultimate control over what goes into their mouths).

"From a toddler's point of view, mealtimes provide a perfect opportunity for practicing all sorts of skills that have nothing to do with food," says Dr. Winchell. "While sitting at the table, picking at their meal, they can learn about manipulation, control, independence, approval, pleasing, and rebellion, for instance. And it's a fairly safe environment to misbehave in, since the short-term consequences [not eating] aren't that severe."

Avoiding Power Struggles

When a two-year-old uses food to annoy you, try not to notice. For one thing, you can't eliminate your child's desire to fight for power and control; in fact, you shouldn't even try. As James Windell points out, "Parents may envision and prefer compliant, easily malleable children. But young children grow into relatively well-behaved older children by being allowed to grow through various stages of developing autonomy."

For another thing, you simply can't win a power struggle with a two-year-old. If your child says *"No!"* and you become determined to make him say yes, you put yourself in the position of having to gradually escalate your threats or punishments until you manage to force him to comply. For instance:

YOU: Honey, eat your peas; they're good for you.

YOUR CHILD: No! Yuck. No like peas.

YOU: If you don't eat them, you can't have any dessert.

YOUR CHILD: Me don't care. No peas.

YOU: Okay, if you don't eat them, no dessert and no book before bed tonight.

YOUR CHILD: (crying by now) No peas!

YOU: That's it: If you don't eat your peas right this minute, you won't get dessert or a book for bed for the rest of the week, and you can't go to Jessica's birthday party tomorrow.

Or you may end up ruining your credibility by pleading with your toddler ("Please, sweetie, just one more bite for your dear old dad") or trying to make him feel guilty ("Mommy's so sad. I cooked those peas especially for you, and now you won't eat them").

"Even if your child eventually eats his peas, you still lose," notes Dr. Winchell, "because you override his internal hunger cues and convey the idea that food can be used as a tool of control."

Your Best Response

As with any toddler misbehaviors, eating-related problems and power struggles are best handled with patience and positive discipline. (See the "Discipline Tip" boxes throughout this chapter.) It also helps if you have solutions to common toddler problems at hand, for use at a moment's notice. That way, you won't have to think creatively when you're feeling so frustrated you want to explode. Here are a few ideas that will help:

• *If your child rejects foods, or eats less than you think he needs*—don't get all bent out of shape. "It doesn't mean your child is rejecting you or your offer of love," notes Dr. Schwartzman. "He's merely rejecting the food you're offering at that moment." And unless he's already severely undernourished, or you aren't sure where his next meal will come from, it's highly unlikely that he'll starve.

"In most cases, when a toddler refuses to eat, there's a good reason," says child psychologist Dr. Susan Bergmann. "And usually, it's that he's not hungry."

Another possibility is that your child is sick. As parent Larry Sienkowicz notes, "I'll never forget the time I coaxed my two-year-old into eating, only to have him throw up his entire meal on my shoulder an hour later. It turned out he had a stomach virus, and couldn't eat for another three days."

So trust your toddler: when he's feeling hungry, you can be sure he'll eat. In fact, he may eat so much that you'll start worrying that he's overeating. When my sons were in the toddler stage, they'd often go days without taking more than two bites from anything on their plates, and then suddenly put away two or three sandwiches at one meal. Other parents report that their toddlers will eat one good meal a day and pick at every other. Believe it or not, both of these eating patterns are normal.

Discipline Tip: Ignoring

There's nothing harder than ignoring a child who's being annoying or irritating at the table. But systematic ignoring is one of the best ways to get a young child to stop misbehaving. As Dr. Garber points out, "You may feel like you're doing absolutely nothing to alter the situation, but consistently acting as though certain behaviors aren't happening can bring astonishing results."

To be effective with ignoring, you must:

1. *Identify the behavior you'd like to eliminate* (for example, demanding more food instead of saying please; banging eating utensils on the table during meals; shaking a spill-proof cup over a plate, so the milk sprinkles onto the meat).
2. *Determine whether you can safely ignore it.* Minor misbehaviors such as food refusals, halfhearted temper tantrums, and whining for extra helpings of dessert can usually be ignored. You should *not*, however, ignore aggressive or harmful behavior

such as throwing food, deliberately breaking things, or throwing violent tantrums.

If you decide you can safely ignore a behavior:

3. *Learn to withdraw your attention completely* when it occurs. Don't look at your child, don't touch her, don't smile in amusement or frown in anger, and don't respond to anything she says. Instead, look away, talk to someone else, turn on the radio, look up at the ceiling, or walk out of the room. "You needn't give your child the cold shoulder," says Dr. Garber, "because that is a form of attention, too. Just become so involved with something else that you don't notice how your child is behaving."
4. *Expect the behavior to get worse at first,* as your child strengthens his efforts to gain your attention. Will yourself not to respond.
5. *Once the behavior stops, find a reason to praise your child for a better behavior* ("I like the way you asked for seconds in such a polite way"). If the misbehavior resurfaces, go into ignoring mode again. "The more consistent you are, and the more completely you remove your attention from the target behavior," adds Dr. Garber, "the sooner it will subside."

• *If your child will eat food only when it's served a certain way*—within reason, try to accommodate her quirky requests. Cut the pizza slice rather than insisting she eat it whole; let her have her morning cereal without milk; use a plate with separate compartments so foods won't touch; let her dip her broccoli in her juice. These kinds of requests are part of your child's desire to feel more in control of her world and her food. They are not eating behaviors that will continue into adulthood, and they do not indicate that your child is spoiled, only normal.

Be aware, however, that accommodating a toddler's requests can be tricky, since two-year-olds often don't know what they really want until you give them something else. "So give it your best shot, but don't go overboard," says Dr. Ayoob. "Your child also needs to know there are limits."

I remember there was a time when I didn't dare make a sandwich for my son without first running down a detailed list of questions: Do you want this bread or that one? Do you want raspberry or strawberry jam? Do you want crunchy or creamy peanut butter? Should I cut the sandwich in rectangles or triangles? Should I cut off the crusts or leave them on? It was a pain in the neck, but it immediately reduced the amount of crying and complaining that accompanied lunch.

However, it didn't completely cure lunchtime tantrums. Sometimes, even after fulfilling all requests with precision, tears still rolled down my child's cheeks because somewhere between the kitchen and the dining table, he had changed his mind. In those cases, I learned to be patient. I didn't run back into the kitchen to try to "fix" things. I simply said: "I'm sorry it isn't the way you'd like it to be. But I can't recut the bread. But if you want, I'll do it differently tomorrow."

"It's fairly typical for young children to make a choice and then change their minds," notes Windell. "And you often can't prevent a tantrum. But if you accept that the behavior—and your child's feelings of indecision and frustration—are normal, it's easier to walk away from such outbursts and let them run their course. If you stay and try to reason with your child, or try to calm him down by giving him what he wants, you end up encouraging more tantrums."

• *If your child wants only one kind of food day after day*—your nutrition radar may start sending out loud, panicky signals. Don't listen. Such food jags are quite common at this age, and seem to have little long-term effect on a child's health or eating habits. "Often, they're a reflection of your child's desire to maintain a comfortable routine in the midst of all the new challenges she's facing," notes Marjorie Sutton, M.S., R.D., L.D., C.S., a pediatric nutrition specialist at the University of Chicago Children's Hospital.

The best way to respond to a food jag is to serve the food your child likes, *along with* other healthful alternatives in case she changes her mind or gets curious about other textures and flavors. "If the food jag is candy, of course, you'll have to set some limits," notes Dr. Ayoob. "But otherwise, there's no reason to fight it." Eventually, all food jags run their course; before you know it, your child will get bored with eating only white bread and rice and move on to a new obsession, like cheese at every meal.

• *If your child rejects the new foods you offer*—keep on offering them. Children this age are much more aware of the world around them; they now know when something is unfamiliar or different, and they rarely like it.

Even foods your child once accepted without question may now be refused because they look or smell "funny" or remind him of "yucky" or "scary" things.

"When he was about two-and-a-half, my son

Thomas went through a stage where he refused to eat anything that didn't have a clean edge to it," recalls Marcy Beyer (not her real name), a mother of two. "For some strange reason, he had decided that anything straggly—like the jagged edge of a bread crust or a strand of cheese falling from his pizza—was a 'scary spider.' Convincing him otherwise was impossible, so I just let things ride. If he was afraid of something on his plate, I took it off without comment. Eventually—thank goodness—the spider phase passed."

Toddlers' food allegiances shift and change, so you shouldn't be discouraged by one rejection, says Corinne Montandon. "In fact, the more often a child sees a food, the more likely she is to eventually taste it."

Discipline Tip: Making "No" Sound Like "Yes"

One of the easiest ways to start a fight with a two-year-old is to use the word no. So, whenever possible (when safety is not the issue), try to say yes to your child, even if your real answer is no. That doesn't mean lying; it means phrasing your vetoes in a positive way. For example:

* If your child starts whining for a cookie before dinner, say: *"Sure, you can have a cookie—when it's time to eat dinner."*
* If he's bugging you to play blocks with him, but you have to put supper on the table, say: *"I'll be happy to play blocks with you—as soon as I'm finished cooking. Why don't you start getting the blocks set up while I cook?"*
* If she ignores your requests to come eat lunch because

she wants to watch a video, say: *"Great idea! We'll pick out a video now—so we can watch it as soon as we finish our lunch."*

- If he starts complaining because you served chicken instead of macaroni and cheese, say: *"I like macaroni and cheese, too—let's plan to have some tomorrow."*
- If she starts crying because she wants an orange Popsicle and you're fresh out, say: *"We're out of orange Popsicles—but you can pick grape or strawberry instead."*

• *If your child throws a tantrum over food*—try not to react in kind. Temper tantrums are very common at this age, so you shouldn't be surprised if your child tries throwing a few over food. They can happen for any reason: because you won't give your child a bag of chips before dinner; you give her a cookie, but it breaks; you take away her milk because she's spilling it; she doesn't like what you're having for dinner; she doesn't want to sit in her high chair; she wants to use her blue cup instead of her purple one; she wants to feed herself but can't get the food on her spoon.

There are different ways of handling toddler tantrums, depending on why they're being thrown and how your child is acting. In general, the best approach is to follow these steps:

1. First, try to ignore the tantrum. If your child is throwing it because she wants another cup of milk, and you're in the process of refilling her cup anyway, tell her, "When we want milk in this house, we say, 'Please may I have more milk in a nice voice.'" Then finish what you're doing and hand her the cup.

If she's screaming for something you *don't* think she should have—like a breakable glass she can drop on the floor or a sip of your hot coffee—don't give in. Your child needs to learn that certain behaviors are simply unacceptable, and no amount of fussing or crying will change your mind. Just say, "I'm sorry you're upset, but I can't give you a sip of my coffee because it's too hot and it might burn your mouth. Coffee is for grown-ups. Can I get you some milk or juice instead?"

If the tantrum continues, turn your attention away from your child. Most outbursts occur for the sole purpose of gaining an adult's attention. If you can resist reacting, the tantrum will dissipate of its own accord.

2. If you can't ignore the tantrum—it occurs at the dinner table or you're in a public eating area—try distraction. Many two-year-olds will quickly forget about crying and complaining if you give them something else more interesting to do, like pull paper off a straw, listen to the way you can crunch on your celery, count carrots, look out the window, or sing the alphabet song.

3. If distraction doesn't work, remove your child from the dinner table and put her into a chair, her bedroom, or another quiet place for some cool-down time. Tell her in a calm voice that she can't return to the table until she's finished with her tantrum. If she's so out of control she's in danger of hurting herself or breaking something, simply hold her firmly but gently until the outburst is over. Do not talk to her while she's in cool-down time, and above all, do not try to reason with her. You can stay nearby, or if you're holding her, gently repeat a soothing phrase such as, "We'll go back to the table as soon as you calm down." But don't engage her in any other conversation; don't respond to her accusa-

tions or pleas; don't even look her in the eye until she's quiet.

4. As soon as she's regained her composure, let her return to the table and carry on as though nothing happened. Lecturing your child about her misbehavior or her tantrum won't help at this point, and it may trigger another outburst. You can always talk about good table manners at another time. (For a more in-depth discussion of tantrum behaviors and how to manage them, consult *Tantrums: Secrets to Calming the Storm,* another book in the *Child* Magazine parenting series.)

--------------------- ✳ ---------------------

Discipline Tip: Distracting

Meeting a stubborn toddler head-on is like throwing a lit match into a pool of lighter fluid. A better approach when you want to change an undesirable behavior is distraction: quickly finding something else for your child to think about or do.

For instance, say you've just served your toddler some apple slices, and he starts crying because he wants peaches (which you don't have). Rather than respond to him in frustration or anger ("That's all we've got, so you have to eat it!"), explain calmly that you're out of peaches and then quickly shift his attention elsewhere. For instance, you could:

◆ Hum his favorite nursery tune;
◆ Say, "Oh, look out the window! There's a big red truck passing by!";
◆ Talk about what you plan to do when breakfast is over

("I can't wait till we've finished eating so we can read our new library book together");

♦ Ask your child a question ("Can you guess what my favorite color is?");

♦ Move him to another area for a change in scenery ("Let's eat our lunch on the porch so we can enjoy the flowers").

Kids this age tend to have short memories, and they rarely hold a grudge. So if you can get your child's mind off peaches, he won't even notice he's eating apple slices instead.

• *If your child wants to eat dessert first*—let him. That doesn't mean allowing him to fill up on sweets, or to eat as much dessert as his tiny tummy can handle. It means putting a small amount of dessert at his place along with the rest of his meal, and letting him eat his food in whatever order he pleases.

Another option, according to Mary Abbott Hess, is to let your child know that dessert is part of the meal, no matter what. "I believe that serving dessert after dinner is important because that's how most people in our society eat, so it's part of teaching socialization skills," she explains. "But you can still reduce the value of dessert by making it clear that even if your child only pushes his other foods around the plate, when dessert is served at the end of the meal, he can still have a small piece."

If you were brought up to think of dessert as a treat at the end of the meal that only came if you actually ate the rest of your meal, you may find this advice somewhat shocking. But according to the experts, it makes sense for a number of reasons:

1. It puts sweets on an equal par (emotionally) with meats, breads, fruits, vegetables, and other healthier foods. "If your child can freely alternate bites of cookie with bites of his sandwich or his salad, he's not likely to think of sweets as a prize for good behavior," notes Sanna James, M.S., R.D., a registered dietitian based in Mill Valley, California, and editor of *Tiny Tummies Nutrition News*, a newsletter for parents. "Instead, he'll accept them as one of the many good things he finds on his plate." Or, if he knows he's going to get the dessert no matter what, then he's not likely to rush through his meal so he can get "the prize," or whine for "the good food" all during the meal.

"However," says Mary Abbott Hess, "to make this strategy work, you need to make it clear that the portion of dessert you're serving is all he gets." In other words, there are no seconds on desserts—even if he throws a tantrum, refuses to eat anything else on his plate, or gobbles up everything else and asks for more dessert. "You should also store any remaining dessert out of sight," Hess adds.

2. It encourages children not to overeat just to get dessert. We've all heard (and most of us have said) things like, "No ice cream until you finish your chicken." But rather than ensure that our kids get proper nutrition, that approach actually encourages them to overeat ("Hmm," the child thinks, "I'm really full, but if I can stuff in a few more bites of chicken, I'll get to have some ice cream!"). This, in turn, dulls a child's sensitivity to what his own stomach is saying: "You're full. Stop eating! Have the ice cream later."

3. It gives your child one less thing to argue about. Kids have an amazing ability to figure out what will

push their parents' buttons. If your toddler senses that dessert is something special, he'll use it as a bargaining chip or battle ax whenever and however he can ("So, you want me to stay quiet during dinner . . . then hand over the candy bar right now"). But if it's there on his plate, and he can eat it or not eat it as he chooses, there's nothing to be gained by whining or begging.

• *If your child wants to mix his foods in strange ways*—let him. I've seen my kids do all sorts of weird things, like dipping their cookies in chicken noodle soup, or adding grapes to a ham sandwich. It turns my stomach, but it doesn't seem to affect their appetites. "Touching and experimenting with food is just another way in which young children explore their taste buds and learn to feel comfortable with their food," notes Dr. Ayoob.

Of course, if the habit extends to wasting lots of food (as in, "Mom, I dumped my ice cream on my spaghetti and it doesn't taste good anymore, so can I have some more ice cream?"), you should set some limits. For instance, before it happens you can say: "If you really want to, you can dump your ice cream onto your spaghetti, but if you don't like it, I can't give you more of those foods. It's your decision."

• *If your child wants to eat with his fingers*—let him. Even if he can eat comfortably with a spoon or fork, he may prefer his fingers for certain foods, or he may find that when he's really hungry he can't eat quickly enough with a spoon or fork. "Allowing him to decide the best method for eating is part of encouraging his budding independence," notes Dr. Ayoob. "It also re-assures him that he has some control over what goes into his mouth." As he gets older and more competent with utensils, simple reminders ("We eat our cereal with a spoon") should be sufficient to guide his behavior.

• *If your once-competent child asks you to feed him*—indulge his whim. Even when young children can eat with a fork and spoon, they sometimes get the urge to be fed like babies again. It's part of their struggle to separate and remain attached at the same time.

There's no need to worry that your child is regressing or to insist that he use his hard-won skills at all times. He can slip a bit and have you feed him once or twice without risking a total backslide. Eventually, if you don't make too big a deal of it, his desire to move and grow will triumph over his desire to be treated like a baby again. In the meantime, he'll move on to the next stage of development feeling more confident than ever that you'll always be there when he needs you.

"Another thing I often see is young children who won't touch what's on their plates, but will eat off Mom or Dad's," notes Dr. Ayoob. "That's okay to me—as long as they're getting a balanced diet from their parents' plates. The habit of eating a balanced healthy meal will eventually transfer over: your child will not be asking to eat from your plate when he's thirteen."

• *If your toddler finishes eating before the rest of the family*—allow him to leave the table. "While some two-year-olds can sit through an entire meal, many cannot," says Dr. Winchell. In fact, most kids this age have trouble sitting through a whole episode of *Barney*, which is far more entertaining than food. So don't expect your toddler to sit and wait after he's had his fill. Let him leave the table and play quietly as the rest of the family finishes their meal (but keep the TV off).

"If he leaves the table and then keeps running back for another bite, make it clear that if he wants to eat he has to sit down," says Dr. Winchell. If he leaves the table and then starts distracting other family members, focus your energies on ignoring his bids for attention.

"When our two-year-old, Luke, leaves the table, and then tries to come back and get us to play with him, we tell him we can't play because we're still eating," says Holly DeGregori, a mother of two. "Sometimes, if he's persistent, my husband will say something funny like, 'Nope, I can't get up. There's glue on my bottom!' Then Luke will just laugh and run off to play."

• *If your child dawdles with his food*—be patient. Most young children are experts at dawdling, and it usually drives their parents crazy. But it's not meant to. As James Windell explains, "Toddlers operate on their own time schedule, and most need at least twice as much time to do things as grown-ups do."

Rather than get annoyed, build in extra time for your child to eat. If she lingers on long after everyone else has finished, or you're in a particular hurry, use a timer to speed your child up, as in, "We need to finish up lunch so we can get to Grandma's on time. I'll set the timer for ten more minutes, and when the buzzer goes off, we'll clean up our mess and go."

That way, if your child gets upset, you can sidestep a power struggle by explaining, "I'm sorry, honey, but the buzzer says it's time to go."

✳

Discipline Tip: Managing Yourself

Patience is more than just a virtue when it comes to raising a strong-willed child: it's a necessity. As Rex Forehand, Ph.D., and Nicholas Long, Ph.D., point out in their book *Parenting the Strong-Willed Child,* "Strong-willed children respond best to parents who can handle problems in a matter-of-fact way. When you lose your patience, you not only set a bad example, you lose control of effectively managing your child's behavior."

To increase your patience level, learn to look at your child's behavior in a more positive way, advises Dr. Forehand. In particular, try to avoid:

+ Thinking in absolute terms, with words like *should, always,* or *never* (as in, "My child *should* eat his vegetables"; "He *always* acts like an animal at the table"; and "He *never* likes what I cook"). Instead, use words like *could, sometimes,* and *some day will;*
+ Ascribing adult motives (such as cruelty and revenge) to your child's misbehavior ("She won't eat because she's angry at me"; "She knew I was having a bad day and she spilled her milk anyway");
+ Taking his actions too personally ("I must be a terrible parent, since my child never eats").

  Instead, frequently tell yourself things like:

+ "All children misbehave at times, even when they know the rules."
+ "While it is undesirable and irritating when my child misbehaves, it is not the end of the world, and it doesn't mean I'm a failure at parenting."
+ "Getting angry at my child will scare him and set a bad example, but it won't help his behavior improve."
+ "My child does not misbehave to make me suffer, but to test her own abilities and boundaries."

——————————— ✳ ———————————

• *If your child wants to snack all day*—don't encourage it. While frequent small meals are good for kids, all-day grazing is not. "The solution is to schedule three daily snack breaks in between meals, so your child has the opportunity to eat every two or three hours," advises Marjorie Sutton. Then you can respond to ill-timed food requests with a matter-of-fact comment like: "Oh, the clock says it's not snack time yet."

This doesn't mean you should be totally rigid about snacks. If your child doesn't normally ask for handouts all day, don't worry if she occasionally requests an unscheduled snack. She's probably going through a growth spurt and needs the extra calories. Or if you're out doing errands and you know lunch or dinner will be delayed, there's no harm in offering an unscheduled snack to keep your child from becoming ravenous and out of control.

AGE FLAG: 3 TO 5 YEARS

MOVING TOWARD CIVILIZED EATING

For many parents, a child's third birthday brings a sigh of relief. Not because they're free and clear of the oppositional behavior their child exhibited in the two-year-old stage, but because they see more and more glimmers of what having a civilized child is like.

It's not just that the preschool-age child is more physically mature and experienced than the toddler. The real benefits come from the fact that around ages three and four, kids become more skilled at expressing their emotions and opinions with words rather than actions. So instead of throwing food or throwing tantrums when they don't like what you serve them, they become more likely to tell you. And even better, they can listen, understand, and respond more appropriately when you explain why their behavior is unacceptable.

Three-year-olds are also much more interested in pleasing their parents than toddlers are. As James Windell notes, "The average three-year-old would rather imitate his parents than oppose them. Therefore, he is easier to manage and much more conforming. He will tend to be more loving and affectionate, and in general more on the delightful side than not."

Focus on Manners

For all of these reasons, three is the perfect age to begin teaching table manners, according to Carol McD. Wallace, author of *Elbows off the Table, Napkin in the Lap, No Video Games during Dinner: The Modern Guide to Teaching Children Good Manners*. But don't expect this task to be quick or easy. "The kinds of eating-related manners that civilized Western society expects don't come naturally to most children," says Wallace. "Nor does the habit of thinking about what would be helpful, kind, or convenient to other people. Teaching manners is a long-term project."

"It shouldn't be your goal to produce a perfectly behaved three-year-old," she adds. "Instead, aim for having a twelve-year-old who's not painful to sit next to at the dinner table."

Where should you begin? According to Wallace, sometime between ages three and five, you can introduce the concepts of:

• Staying seated at the table (for at least ten minutes);
• Sitting in the chair (as opposed to standing on it);

- Waiting for others to be seated before beginning to eat;
- Not talking with food in your mouth;
- Keeping your mouth closed while chewing;
- Not eating with your fingers;
- Using utensils correctly;
- Not waving utensils around;
- Not playing with food;
- Not shoveling food into an already full mouth;
- Eating off your own plate;
- Not complaining that the food is yucky;
- Using a napkin instead of your shirt;
- Keeping elbows off the table;
- Keeping your free hand in your lap;
- Not singing at the table;
- Asking to be excused;
- Clearing your place when you're done eating.

Obviously, you can't introduce all of these concepts at once. Instead, ignore whatever behaviors are merely annoying or irritating to you (such as eating with fingers or humming instead of eating), and start setting limits on the one or two you simply can't accept (such as throwing food at other family members, taking food from the table and eating in another room, or screaming and hitting during a meal).

"Also, make sure your child is developmentally ready for whatever you propose," says Wallace. If he doesn't have the dexterity to use a fork without stabbing himself in the eye, there's no point in insisting he use a fork to eat meat. Wait until his coordination improves.

How to Teach Manners

It usually takes more than one trick to get a new table rule established. According to Carol McD. Wallace, setting a good example comes first: "Modeling the behavior you want your child to emulate is the single most powerful thing you can do to teach him anything," she explains. Other effective tools include:

• *Praise.* But don't just hand out random praise, such as: "You're so wonderful"; "You're the best-behaved boy in town"; or "What a great eater you are." Be specific and describe the actions that meet your approval. For instance, "I like the way you asked politely to be excused"; "I notice you're being very careful to use your napkin instead of your shirt when you wipe your face"; and "It was thoughtful of you to wait until everyone sat down before eating."

"For preschool children, specific, descriptive praise is extremely important," says Dr. Forehand. "The more information and feedback you can provide, the sooner they'll learn the appropriate behaviors."

One thing you shouldn't praise, however, is *how much* your child eats. Eating a lot should occur only because your child is hungry, not because she's trying to please you. Eating a little should also reflect her hunger, not some misguided desire to stay thin or lose weight or even eat healthy. Kids this age are far too young to be worrying about things like that, and restrictive diets may put them at nutritional risk. So save your praise for eating behaviors and table manners, instead of appetite and consumption.

• *Practice.* "Every now and then, we play a game

called Good Manners with our children," says Katy Musolino, a mother of two. "We talk ahead of time about the kinds of behaviors that qualify as good manners, and then when we sit at the table, we all try to outdo each other in polite table behaviors. The kids love it because they think it's a game." Other parents engage in special tea parties with their kids, or make a game of practicing good manners when going out to eat. Special dress-up meals on holidays and other special occasions will also further the cause.

• *Prompting.* As Carol McD. Wallace puts it, "A stream of gentle, courteous reminders, sometimes known as nagging, is essential."

James Windell agrees. "Stating a rule once does not guarantee that a child will remember or obey it," he explains. "In fact, most young children need to have rules repeated often, because they forget them." It's partly because they have so many rules to learn at this stage, and partly because there are so many other interesting things in the world to distract them.

So don't get angry if you have to tell your child over and over and over again to swallow his food before he talks, or use his napkin. "When a child forgets a rule it doesn't mean he's evil, spiteful, rebellious, or destined for a life of delinquency," says James Windell. "All it means is that a rule was temporarily forgotten. It's your job to remind him."

But don't overdo it or get nasty; children tend to eat poorly when they face a constant stream of criticism or correction at the table.

• *Punishment.* For seriously bad manners, you can also employ consequences (as in, "If you throw your food again, you'll have to leave the table and sit in your room for two minutes"). Make sure the consequences you set are fair, reasonable, and enforceable. And after giving a fair warning, be sure you follow through with whatever you promised without getting angry or upset ("You threw your food again. I'm putting you in your room and setting the timer for two minutes"). Otherwise, your child will learn to push and push until you explode.

OTHER WAYS TO HELP

As you work on teaching your child table manners, keep in mind that your ultimate goal is to make eating a pleasant, pressure-free activity. If any of the problem behaviors we talked about in the two-year-old section emerge, handle them in the same way (see pages 114 to 121), without allowing yourself to get too worked up or angry. Otherwise, concentrate on:

• *Helping your child feel more grown up.* Once he's big enough to sit in a real chair instead of a high chair, let him (use a booster seat if necessary). If he asks to use an adult-size spoon and fork, put away his toddler tools. Once he can eat with some degree of neatness, exchange his bib for a napkin tucked under his chin. Your child is much more likely to imitate the eating habits of the adults around him if he's encouraged to feel like a big boy.

However, don't push your child beyond his skill level. If he still can't handle a cup without a spill-proof lid, don't offer one when he's really hungry; if he still tends to slobber all over the place, keep him well supplied with bibs (find some that don't have babyish designs); if cups and plates have a habit of slipping from his hands, don't give him anything breakable. He should feel challenged enough to remain self-confident but not overwhelmed.

• *Eating at least one meal a day together as a family.* In today's fast-paced world, it's amazingly easy to go through an entire day or longer without ever sitting down together as a family. And it's tempting, when you have young children in the house, to schedule your own dinner for after the kids are in bed, to avoid the stress of eating with them. But "sitting down at a table that's been set with some degree of care is an important part of teaching young children what civilized dining is all about," says Marjorie Sutton. "It's also an important opportunity for you to model proper eating behaviors." (Plus, according to one study of 270,000 children, it's an important factor in success at school.)

In addition to eating together regularly (if once a day isn't realistic, try for several times a week), try to schedule some more formal dinners with your child to help him practice the finer dining skills he'll need when eating at restaurants or at other people's homes for special occasions. This will also help him see that eating is more than just a chance to refill his tummy, but a social experience that can be rich and enjoyable. Little touches such as special plates, cloth napkins, flowers on the table, and special drinks can make even an ordinary meal seem like a special occasion.

✳

Discipline Tip: Time-Out

If your child isn't in the mood to listen to your rules, the best response is time-out (removing her from the table and making her sit in a boring place for a few minutes, until she's ready to behave). Unlike other punishments such as yelling and spanking, which give a child negative attention, time-out works by withdrawing attention completely. "The removal of attention can be just as effective as most forms of punishment, without the negative side effects," notes Dr. Forehand.

As he points out in his book, *Parenting the Strong-willed Child*, the first step in using time-out effectively, is to choose a time-out location. Try to make sure it is nowhere near any pleasant distractions such as toys, windows, the TV, or people. Your best bet is a hallway, a kitchen corner, or a chair in your bedroom (it's probably more boring than your child's bedroom!). However, never use a scary place such as a closet, basement, bathroom, or other dark or dangerous room. Your goal is not to terrify your child, but to make her miss your positive attention.

Once you've designated a time-out spot, explain to your child that she'll be sent there when she misbehaves, and she'll need to stay there until she's ready to behave again.

Then, when a misbehavior occurs:

1. Remind your child of whatever family rule she's breaking (for example, "We do not stand in our chairs while we're eating").
2. If she keeps acting up, issue a warning ("If you don't sit down, you'll have to sit in time-out").
3. If the warning is ignored, tell her she's in time-out ("You didn't sit down, so you're now in time-out"). She may try to immediately comply with the family rule, but at this point, it's better to go ahead with the time-out. Otherwise, she'll get in the habit of pushing

you to the limits of your patience before she com-
plies.

4. Lead (or if necessary, carry) your child to the time-out
location without talking, lecturing, reasoning, explaining, arguing, or yelling. She may cry, kick,
scream, or beg for another chance. She may even
tell you that you're a horrible parent, she's going to
run away, and she hates you. Don't listen and don't
respond. You must remain neutral.

5. When she's in the right place, set a timer for three or
four minutes (usually, one minute per year of child's
age) and let her know she's in time-out until the timer
rings. Then, turn or walk away. *Do not give her any
attention*, not even eye contact. If she gets out of the
time-out spot, lead her back and reset the timer; if
necessary, stand behind her with your hands on her
shoulders to encourage her to stay put. Do not start
the timer until your child is where she should be.

6. When the timer rings, check to see if your child is
quiet. If she's still kicking and screaming, reset the
timer; if she's quiet, tell her briefly that time-out is over
and let her know she can return to the table if she's
ready to follow the rules ("You can come to the table
now, if you're finished standing in your seat"). If
she's not calm, and not ready to comply, reset the
timer; repeat the process until she's ready to behave.

Last but not least, don't expect time-out to work immediately, or to eliminate a misbehavior altogether.
It's most effective in defusing misbehavior and prevent-
ing parent/child power struggles. Over time, however, if used consistently, it can also act as a deterrent
(as in, "If you do that again, you'll be in time-out").

———————— ✳ ————————

OUTSIDE INFLUENCES

There's one more eating challenge you should prepare for in the preschool years: peer pressure. "As your child becomes more socially active—going to play dates, preschool, and other activities outside the home—and more aware of television ads, he's going to be exposed to different types of food and different rules about eating," notes Mary Abbott Hess. Some of the foods and rules will be things you don't approve of, and some of the snacks he receives at preschool and at other people's homes will make you fear that all your efforts toward healthy eating are doomed.

I remember showing up at my son's preschool for a Halloween party and watching in horror as the children were served not only orange-and-black cupcakes, but cookies, cheese twists, chocolate candies, and Kool-Aid. (Talk about a sugar overdose! Even I couldn't put away that much junk food!) Much to my relief, most of the kids were sensible enough to take only a few nibbles of one or two items and then run off to play.

Try not to overreact when your preschooler comes home with a chocolate mustache or a bellyful of foods you would never even buy, much less serve (we'll explain why in Chapter Five). And, if he starts asking for the same kind of lunch his best friend brings to preschool, try to be open-minded, even if it's food you consider junk. This is an age of experimentation and the very beginning of a long passage of peer influences. "But you still have the majority control over what your child eats, so there's no reason to panic," says Hess. Instead, field your child's new food requests with an open mind and optimistic spirit, while continuing to make sure that he gets a balanced diet at home.

✳

Discipline Tip: The Broken-Record Technique

What do you do when you've carefully explained to a child *why* she can't have or do something, and she still whines and complains? Stand your ground without getting angry or giving in, advises Dr. Garber. "There's no point in trying to reason forever with a child who refuses to accept no for an answer," he explains. "If you do, you only encourage your child to use persistent comments and questions ('But why can't I?' or 'You promised!') to wear you down every time she wants to get her own way."

A better technique is to explain your reason once ("You can't eat your apple while you're running around, because you might choke"), and then respond to any additional complaints or demands by calmly repeating one brief statement. For example:

CHILD:	Daddy, I want some apple.
YOU:	No apple until you're sitting down.
CHILD:	Gimme some apple right now!
YOU:	No apple until you're sitting down.
CHILD:	(crying) Why can't I? You promised!
YOU:	No apple until you're sitting down.

"This broken-record technique works best when you also act like you're paying very little attention to your child's additional pleas," says Dr. Garber. "Just continue whatever you're doing, and repeat the phrase in a neutral voice whenever your child tries to engage you."

At the same time, steel yourself for a backlash. "At first, your child may respond by getting angry or throwing a tantrum," says Dr. Garber. "But eventually, his demands and questions will decrease because he'll get tired of hearing the same old answer." If his misbehavior crosses the line into name calling, hitting, or other types of aggression, use time-out or another form of discipline to stop the misbehavior. But don't give in to the initial demand.

5 HOW BIG KIDS EAT

AGE FLAG: 5 TO 6 YEARS

The Easier Years

Once you've survived the toddler and preschool years, the early elementary school years may seem like a breeze. Sure, there are still problems and confrontations. But five- and six-year-olds are so much more rational and self-controlled than two-, three-, and four-year-olds that difficulties and disagreements often seem more logical and easier to handle. Your child can now *tell* you why he's crying or upset, and you can now *explain* why he shouldn't eat chocolate cake for breakfast.

Plus, kids this age are better than ever at:

- Understanding and following rules;
- Helping out with chores and taking on new responsibilities;

- Controlling their emotions;
- Delaying gratification;
- Joining in on mealtime conversations;
- Using a fork and spoon correctly, and with confidence;
- Eating what they like, and asking for seconds—politely—if they're still hungry;
- Saying no to food they don't want, in a polite manner.

All this budding maturity and skill will make life a whole lot easier for you. But it's still too soon to expect perfection. "If a household has exacting standards, the child of this age may still fall short," notes Dr. Louise Bates Ames of the Gesell Institute. "He dawdles, talks too much, may even toward the end of a meal ask to be fed. He wriggles in his chair, though he doesn't as a rule have to leave the table to go to the bathroom as he did at four. And, though appetite is usually improved, food preferences are still rather marked."

Adds James Windell, "Though five- and six-year-olds often seem to be fairly mature when they remember rules and try very hard to please, they are still youngsters, and their growth and development is still subject to both ups and downs." One minute your child may be showing off how big, strong, and independent she is by setting the table or serving her sister breakfast, and the next minute she may be talking like a baby and asking you to feed her. Of if there's a new baby in the house, she may even want to drink from a bottle again.

It's important to be patient with your child during these inevitable moments of regression, whether or not they involve food. For instance, if your child wants to try out a baby bottle, let her. It's unlikely she'll stick with it for very long. But if you insist she's too old or refuse to let her experiment, she may feel left out and resentful. Unless a babyish behavior persists for a long time, there's no harm in indulging your child, or in simply ignoring it. In fact, the less fuss you make, the sooner it's likely to fade away. Children this age generally use temporary regressions to reassure themselves that you're still there for them; that, in turn, gives them the courage to forge ahead with the next big leap in development.

WHAT TO EXPECT

As with younger children, knowing what to expect from your five- or six-year-old can make a big difference in how you react when certain table behaviors occur. For example, if you think your child is refusing food or fidgeting in his chair just to bug you or get attention, you may end up applying unnecessarily harsh or strict punishment. But if you know that those behaviors are common among kids your child's age, you're more likely to focus on guiding your child toward better ways of behaving.

Here then, are some common characteristics of five- and six-year-olds that may affect eating and table behaviors:

FIVE-YEAR-OLDS LOVE TO:

• *Show off.* And they now have the vocabulary and language skills to brag about their accomplishments.

Expect to hear a lot of comments like, "Look how strong I am, I can carry two grocery bags at once"; "I'm so big now I can eat two bowls of cereal for breakfast"; and "I'm really helping you, aren't I?" And don't be afraid to say, "You sure are a big help," or "You really have gotten strong." Your child is proud of his new abilities and accomplishments, and needs to hear that you've noticed them, too. As James Windell notes, "Fives respond well to praise, positive attention, and encouraging feedback." Supporting your child's self-appreciation will build his self-esteem; he can always learn about modesty later on.

• *Help out.* Again, kids this age have the coordination and strength to do more than ever before, as well as a strong desire to cooperate. So this is a great age to get your child involved in kitchen and mealtime chores: setting and clearing the table, helping with menu planning and grocery shopping, even doing some cooking. "The more involved your child is in preparing the food that's served to him, the more open he'll be to eating it," says Dr. Ayoob.

Be aware, however, that your child may overestimate his abilities. He may want to use the sharp knives, for instance, or drink out of your best crystal to prove how grown up he is. Don't be afraid to set limits when you know your child is trying to do too much, even if he protests (as in, "Why not? Jeremy's parents let him!"). Instead, supervise your child closely when he's practicing new skills, and find alternatives if there's a danger of injury or breakage ("You can't use that knife because it's too sharp and heavy, but you can try this one; I'll show you how").

• *Follow routines.* Five-year-olds tend to be less adventurous than fours; they have a better idea of what the boundaries of their world are, and they enjoy living within them. They especially appreciate having a predictable schedule, so it should be fairly easy for you to maintain a regular meal- and snack-time routine. The downside is that your child may rebel or throw a tantrum if the usual eating routine is broken or you inject new elements without warning (giving her a different place mat, for instance, or serving her milk in her usual juice glass). Try to go with the flow when your child cries or complains about these things, and if you know a change in the usual routine is coming, give fair warning ("We'll be eating supper a little later today because we have company coming over"; "I'm putting out paper plates today because our dishwasher is broken").

• *Imitate adults.* How you behave at the dinner table—the way you eat, what you talk about, the foods you eat—will make a greater impression on your five-year-old than what you say about eating and table manners. In other words, if you warn your child not to talk with his mouth full, but you or other family members do it regularly, he's unlikely to stop. So be sure to be on your best behavior and model the kind of eating habits you'd like your child to imitate.

• *Please their parents.* One of the most wonderful things about kids this age is that they genuinely want to please their parents and do the right thing. They have a strong sense of fairness and a healthy respect for rules, so if you set limits that they believe are fair and reasonable, they'll usually go along with what you ask.

You may run into trouble, however, when your child does something he knows is wrong, whether by accident or on purpose. Rather than risk losing his reputation as a child who cooperates, he may tell a lie or exaggerate the truth to avoid trouble. If this happens, there's no need to overreact or start lecturing your child on the evils of lying. As James Windell notes, "It doesn't mean your child is a compulsive liar if he doesn't accept responsibility for a misbehavior. It just means he doesn't want you to get angry at him."

The best way to react is to find a gentle way to help him explain what happened, Windell advises. "You'll have an easier time dealing with the initial misbehavior if you allow your five-year-old to save face," he explains. For instance, instead of yelling, "Who spilled this juice on my new rug?" try, "Tell me how all that juice got onto my new rug." If he tries to shift the blame ("The dog jumped up and knocked it out of my hand"), respond in a nonaccusatory manner: "Next time, please drink your juice in the kitchen or at the table, so if the dog knocks it over it won't stain the rug. Now, how about getting me a damp sponge, so we can clean this up."

＊

Discipline Tip: Setting Consequences

Fairness is a big issue with five- and six-year-olds. So it's more important than ever to be logical and reasonable when setting consequences for misbehavior. "Though popular, spanking, criticizing, threatening, yelling, or embarrassing your child are among the least effective ways to change a behavior," according to Dr. Garber. They may work in the short run, but they won't help your child see you as either fair or reasonable over the long term. In fact, they may make her fear and resent you.

To preserve your good relationship with your child and still enforce table and other rules, opt instead for:

* *Natural consequences*—allowing your child to feel the direct effect of his actions. For instance, if he spills cereal all over the floor because he insisted on pouring it into the bowl himself, then he must clean up the mess; if he's acting silly and drops his fruit-juice bar on the ground, he loses it; if he leaves the table to go play before he's finished eating, he can't come back to eat until the next scheduled meal or snack.
* *Withdrawal of privileges*—temporarily taking away something your child cares about, to reinforce the importance of following family rules. For instance, if he refuses to come to the table when dinner is being served because he's watching TV, he loses the privilege of watching TV before dinner the next day; if he uses his knife inappropriately at the table, he loses the privilege of having a knife at his place setting.
* *Time-out*—putting your child in a boring place until he can calm down and behave more appropriately (see box, page 147). If your child is being silly instead of eating, for example, or crying and carrying on because he doesn't like the food you served, you can put him in time-out until he's ready to sit at the table and eat the foods he does like quietly and calmly.

"Before using any of these techniques, make sure you explain to your child how you will react if a certain behavior occurs," adds Dr. Garber. For instance, "If you leave the table before you're finished eating, I'll clear your place and you'll have to wait until the next meal for more food." Then do exactly as you promised. Otherwise, your child will learn to view your consequences as empty threats.

———————————— ✳ ————————————

SIX-YEAR-OLDS TEND TO BE:

• *Enthusiastic eaters.* According to Dr. Ames, "Many sixes love to eat and may seem to be eating all day long. However, their eyes may be bigger than their stomachs, so they often help themselves to more food than they can actually finish."

They also have a tendency to grab food, and insist on the biggest piece; if someone else gets a larger portion, they may complain bitterly about how unfair you are, and how the whole world is against them. Don't feel bullied by such behavior. If an older sibling gets more food on his plate and your six-year-old complains, explain that he can have seconds once he's finished with his first serving; if you're dividing a dessert between two kids, have one child cut the dessert, and let the other get first pick.

Six-year-olds also tend to have very strong food preferences, and either love or hate what you put on their plates. If you run into trouble with food resistance or refusals, follow the advice in Chapter Four.

• *Highly changeable.* Six-year-olds are more confident, capable, and aware of all that life has to offer them, and they tend to be upbeat and enthusiastic most of the time. But then again, they all have moments when they feel overwhelmed and confused by all the choices and challenges presented to them. That's when you'll see the more stubborn and oppositional side of being six. Your child may decide he wants ham for lunch and then switch to turkey as soon as you serve the ham; he may insist on pouring milk from the carton without your supervision and then blame you angrily if the milk spills (even if you weren't in the room); he may boast about how well he sets the table and then whine and complain when you ask him to do it.

Your child is not trying to be difficult in such moments. Like the indecisive toddler, he's trying to take control of his universe. As James Windell explains, "Unlike five-year-olds, who are intent on pleasing their parents, sixes are more concerned about themselves and the things that go on in their lives. They want everything to go their way, and when it doesn't, they can quickly become stubborn, obstinate, and indecisive." Keeping up with the changing nature of a six-year-old can be difficult for parents, but reacting with anger won't help. Patience is a virtue you must continue to cultivate at this stage of your child's life (see box, page 139).

• *Insecure.* Like five-year-olds, sixes love to talk about how great they are; they also have a tendency to insist they can do certain things they really can't (e.g., "I can cook a whole meal by myself"; "That's easy, I could eat ten ears of corn—a lot more than you!"). Then, if they try to prove they can do it but fail, they melt into hysterical tears.

Again, try to be patient with this behavior. Instead of insisting, "There's no way you could eat that much—you're far too little," be sympathetic. Recognize that your child is feeling powerless in a big, scary world, and humor him: "Wow, that's a lot of corn!" Despite the fact that boasting is annoying, and it may make you fear your child will grow up to be a complete egotist, it's common among six-year-olds, who tend to be an insecure lot.

You needn't try to inflate your child's ego by going along with the boasting, though. If your child starts fishing for compliments, respond with open-ended questions. For example, if she says something like, "I'm the best eater in the house, aren't I?" you can respond, "It seems like that's really important to you— tell me what you think it means to be the best eater in the house?" Or, if you don't know what else to say, simply repeat back to your child what you're hearing her say: "So, it sounds like you feel really proud of yourself for being such a good eater."

• *In love with learning.* This is a good time to get your child involved in cooking and grocery shopping, and start teaching him about the Food Guide Pyramid. There's no need to hammer nutritional facts into his brain or make him afraid about eating too much fat or not enough protein. Just expose him to the notion that different foods work together to create a balanced diet. You might want to hang a copy of the Food Guide Pyramid on the refrigerator door, for example, and now and then refer to it when you're planning meals or lunches together. Your child will need this information as he spends more and more time away from home, making his own food choices.

• *Awkward or offensive at the table.* As Dr. Ames points out, "Don't be surprised if your six-year-old stuffs his mouth, talks with his mouth full, grabs for food, knocks over his milk, dribbles, kicks the chair, teeters back in his chair, and, all too often, even falls off his chair." And don't get upset if he eats at a snail's pace, frequently picks fights with his siblings at the dinner table, or refuses to use his napkin, fork, or spoon. (My six-year-old—the kid who was such a neat eater as a toddler—now prefers eating with his fingers and using his shirt as a napkin.)

Kids this age also have a penchant for using meal-times as an opportunity to annoy their parents and entertain their siblings. For example, they love making strange noises, opening their mouths to show you their chewed-up food, burping loudly, and talking about bodily functions. "You may be inclined to think of this period as the gross-out years, rather than the golden years," says James Windell. But try not to react too strongly. Giving frequent rule reminders and using time-out should keep poor table manners in check, without giving undesirable behavior undue attention.

Above all, when mealtimes in your house feel more like a trip to the zoo than a time to relax and refuel, just keep telling yourself, "My child will one day out-grow this behavior and eat like a civilized human." It may take another ten or so years, of course, but it will happen.

✕ FOUR

Special Challenges: Coping with a Picky Eater

With her bright blue eyes and shiny blond hair, five-year-old Whitney Hughes is the picture of health. She's active, energetic, and full of life—but her mother Samantha sometimes wonders where she gets her get-up-and-go. "The child never eats," says Samantha. "When she was younger, she'd go two or three days without eating anything that resembled a meal. And when she did get hungry, she'd eat the same thing, over and over again.

"Once she went on a two-month string-bean binge," Samantha says. "That's all she'd eat for breakfast, lunch, and dinner. I was so worried that I called the pediatrician, but he said to trust her body to know what it needs. Eventually, she did get over it," adds Samantha, "but then all she'd eat was spaghetti." Her latest obsession? Apple-butter sandwiches and Yahoo chocolate drink.

"I keep offering different foods," says Samantha

"but she's very picky. Sometimes I wonder how she can live on so little."

Larry Sienkowicz wonders the same thing about his three-year-old, Aaron. "My son won't eat anything that looks even remotely unusual," he says. "Once I served him a peanut butter and jelly sandwich—his all-time favorite food—and forgot to cut off the crusts, and he wouldn't touch it because he thought it was a different kind of sandwich. I have no idea how the kid survives."

The Result of Frustration

If you have a child who eats like Whitney or Aaron, you're probably feeling as frustrated and anxious as Samantha and Larry. And, like many parents of picky eaters, you may be trying all sorts of tricks to cure your child of this awful-seeming affliction, such as:

- Waking her up at night to feed her;
- Offering snacks every fifteen or twenty minutes during the day;
- Talking about children in other parts of the world who are starving;
- Using desserts to get her to eat healthier foods;
- Forcing her to sit at the table until she cleans her plate; or
- Picking up the spoon or fork and using games, pleading, or funny noises to trick her to open wide and take a bite.

The basic fears fueling such attempts to get a reluctant eater to eat are varied. Some parents worry that their picky eater is either sick or starving himself; others attribute their child's food refusals to their own incompetency at parenting (or cooking); and still others fear that their child will suffer delayed development or end up being too short or too skinny owing to a lack of food. "When you feel responsible for someone else's health and growth, it's hard not to worry when he just pushes the food around his plate," notes Dr. Stephen Garber. "You think you have to do *something* to make sure he gets the nutrition he needs."

The News You Need

What many well-meaning parents don't realize is that nearly all children go through phases when they're finicky about food. "Some children who are extra sensitive to taste and odor are always picky about their food," notes Dr. Dori Winchell. "But even those who usually eat well often go through temporary phases when they suddenly get fussy. It occurs naturally, as their taste buds, bodies, and emotions develop."

However, most picky eaters do not end up undernourished. Even children who seem to eat very little are usually consuming the exact amount of calories and nutrients their little bodies need.

In some cases, of course, picky eating can indicate a serious medical or emotional condition. But for most children under age six, food refusals and strong food preferences are part of growing up. They're not necessarily problem behaviors—unless a parent thinks they are.

"The real problem with picky eating is that it upsets

parents," says Felicia Busch. "They get so worried about their child's health that they become over-involved in what their kid eats. But the more they try to convince their child to eat, the worse the picky eating usually becomes." That's partly because kids don't like to be forced to eat; but it's also because they do like attention—and as soon as they realize that not eating gets it, food refusals can become chronic.

"The best way to keep a child's finicky food habits from getting out of hand," adds Busch, "is to let go of your stress and accept them as normal."

Dr. Dorothy Sendelbach agrees. "I've been through the picky-eater toddler stage three times with my own children, and the only way I survived each time was by convincing myself not to worry."

This chapter will help you stop worrying, too.

<hr>

*

<hr>

When to Call the Doctor

Your child is eating very little (or nothing) *and:*

* Has symptoms of illness, such as fever, chills, ear pain, vomiting, diarrhea, or dehydration;
* Appears to be in pain;
* Has urine that is dark and strong-smelling;
* Doesn't urinate for a whole day;
* Has an abdomen that feels hard or is protruding;
* Shows a sudden loss of weight or drop in appetite;
* Seems unusually tired, listless, or irritable;
* Is under twelve months old and has not gained weight in two months;

* Is over twelve months old and has not gained weight in six months;
* Tends to gag on or throw up certain foods;
* Has been punished by someone for not eating;
* Has not been examined by a doctor in more than a year;
* Is under an unusual amount of stress at home or at school;
* Shows signs of being anxious or depressed.

1 PICKY BABIES

AGE FLAG: 4 TO 12 MONTHS

REASONS FOR FOOD REFUSALS

As your baby grows, there are bound to be times when she rejects regularly scheduled breast milk or formula feedings, or consumes a mere fraction of her usual amount. Once she gets going on solid foods, she may have days when she simply refuses to eat or turns up her nose at previously loved foods. "These temporary rejections can be alarming, but in most cases with children this young, they have a specific cause and are short-lived," notes Dr. Ayoob.

Here are some of the most common causes of food refusals (with tips on how to respond):

• *Sickness:* Illness and eating make terrible companions. A stuffy nose due to a cold, for instance, can make breathing and nursing at the same time difficult;

a stomach or other type of virus can seriously under-mine a child's appetite; and ear pain is often inflamed by the act of sucking. If your baby has thrush (a fungal infection in her mouth) or a sore throat, she may find it too painful to swallow anything.

If sickness is the problem: Trust your baby when she refuses to eat. Forcing food in usually results in spitting it back out. But fluids are important, so ask your pedia-trician how to keep those up, based on your child's age and illness. As soon as your baby starts feeling better, her appetite will return on its own, and she'll probably eat ravenously for a few days to make up for any lost weight.

• *Teething:* Gums swollen due to sprouting teeth may cause pain when your baby tries to bite, suck, or swallow. Typically, a teething baby will act like she's hungry, and ask for food on and off all day, but then turn away quickly each time you feed her, because her mouth pain is greater than her hunger. As soon as the teething pain subsides, your child's normal eating hab-its will resume.

If teething is the problem: Serve cold drinks and chilled foods (for example, icy cold water, a frozen bagel or banana, frozen yogurt or chilled applesauce) to ease the teething pain; offer a cup instead of a bottle; let your child suck on an ice cube wrapped securely in a cloth; let your child chew on a teething biscuit. (However, be sure to supervise your child whenever she's mouthing anything hard or frozen, to prevent choking.)

• *Frustration:* If the hole in the nipple of your child's bottle is too small or is clogged, or the milk isn't flowing from your breasts quickly enough to satisfy his hunger, your baby may turn away in anger and frustration. He may also lose interest in eating if you frustrate him by:

—forcing him to continue nursing (or finish a bottle) when he's no longer hungry;

—frequently jiggling your baby's bottle, adjusting his position, or burping him while he's trying to suck; or

—allowing someone he doesn't know well to feed him, without first briefing that person on how he likes to be fed.

If frustration is the problem: Eliminate the source. That usually means making minor adjustments, such as enlarging the nipple hole of your baby's bottle, trying a different style of nipple, or hand-expressing some milk before you put your baby to your breast. Also, learn to read your baby's hunger and fullness cues; never force him to finish a bottle or nurse longer than he wants to. If he's drinking contentedly, let him be. If someone new is to feed your baby, try to give both of them time to get to know each other first, and be sure to explain the details of how your baby likes to be held, how he likes the bottle held, and how often he needs to be burped.

• *A sensitive temperament:* Some babies are more sensitive to taste, texture, and odor than others. If breast-fed, these children will often balk if their mother eats certain foods with spicy or strong flavors, such as garlic or onions (which can alter the taste of breast milk). Or if the mother is undergoing hormone changes owing to a new pregnancy or the return of menstruation, a sensitive baby might react to the new taste of the milk with a firm refusal to drink it.

Highly sensitive bottle-fed babies sometimes show a preference for the flavor of one type of formula over another. When solid food is introduced, they often require more than the usual amount of time and exposure to accept new foods.

Children with highly sensitive temperaments may also act finicky if:

—they think their milk or food is too hot or too cold;

—you use a new type of bottle, nipple, spoon, or bowl;

—they think the room temperature is too hot or too cold; or

—there are loud or distracting noises during the meal.

If your child has a sensitive temperament: Try to accommodate your baby as much as you can without becoming totally enslaved to her demands. For instance, if you're breast-feeding and she's sensitive to certain things you eat, try not to eat them; if you're bottle feeding, stick with the type of formula you know she prefers; when she starts solids, always put something you know she likes on her plate. Introduce new foods very slowly, using itsy-bitsy portions at first, and don't make a fuss if something isn't eaten or sampled right away. Also, wait until one new food is accepted before presenting another. Always strive for a low-key feeding environment, and whenever possible, buy extras of whatever kind of bottle, cup, bowl, and other feeding equipment your child prefers.

• *An active nature:* Some babies are so active, energetic, and curious about the world that they don't want to spare the time to slow down and eat.

If you have an especially active baby: Take extra

care in making sure the feeding environment is quiet and devoid of enticing toys and other visual distractions. Find out what works best to calm your child down (listening to music, looking at a picture book, taking a ride in the backpack or stroller) and schedule those activities to relax her just before meals.

• *Lack of hunger:* Like adults, babies are hungrier on some days and at some meals than they are at others. As Dr. Garber points out, "It is perfectly normal for a child's appetite to fluctuate from meal to meal, day to day, or even month to month."

If you can't figure out why your child isn't eating: and she doesn't seem to be sick, teething, or experiencing any of the other problems we mentioned—don't worry. She's probably just not feeling hungry. Stick with your usual mealtime schedule so the food will be there when her stomach finally starts growling.

PREVENTION STRATEGIES

The older your baby gets, the more finicky he's likely to become. In addition to following the feeding tips outlined in Chapters Two and Three, there are a number of things you can do now to discourage picky eating later on:

1. *Make sure the foods you serve keep pace with your child's development.* "If you keep your child on strained and pureed baby foods for too long, it can encourage picky eating later on," notes Felicia Busch. "As soon as your child is swallowing well and seems ready to explore different textures [for example, finely minced foods, by around eight to ten months; chopped

foods by ten to twelve months], you should move her forward."

2. *Encourage your baby to touch and mouth things* that are edible, as well as things that are inedible. "Infants learn a great deal about different tastes and textures just by putting things in their mouths and sucking on them," notes Busch. "There's no need to discourage mouthing unless your baby has picked up something that's filthy, poisonous, or unsafe."

3. *Encourage your child to feed herself.* "Most children—if allowed to—can start feeding themselves finger foods by around seven months, and feed themselves completely by about fifteen months," says Mary Abbott Hess. "By the time your child can feed himself for about ten minutes straight, it's time to turn almost all eating responsibility over to him."

Dr. Schmitt agrees. "The greatest tendency among parents of children with poor appetites is to pick up the spoon, load it with food, smile, and try to trick or coerce the child into opening her mouth." It's far better for the child if you encourage her to feed herself as soon as it's clear she can. When she's hungry, she'll eat.

4. *Keep food servings small.* "Many parents think that if they give their child a lot of food, it's like giving a lot of love," says Felicia Busch. "But most young children don't feel loved when they see large portions of food; they feel intimidated by—and resentful of—your high expectations of what they can eat, and they lose their appetite." With most picky eaters, the smaller the initial portion, the better.

5. *Resist the urge to react when your child rejects food.* If a friend were coming to dinner and you knew

he didn't like mushrooms, would you cook a dish that was filled with them? If you noticed during the meal that he had politely pushed the olives in his salad to the side, would you mention it?

Probably not. So why should you treat your picky child any differently? Children are even more tied to their sensory assessments of foods than adults are. And they're more enslaved to their active imaginations. Many, in fact, will reject a food simply because there are spices in the sauce that look like bugs; the color or shape of the food reminds them of ghosts or scary monsters; or something on the plate smells "like a dead guy."

Try to learn to live with the often outrageous reactions your child has to different foods. "Think in terms of 'My child won't eat this particular food *today*,'" says Marjorie Sutton. "He may just love it next week, next month, or next year."

6. *Don't bribe your child to eat or praise her for eating.* We covered this in other chapters, but it's especially important for picky eaters. Studies show that children are more likely to develop new tastes and eat well when they feel free to discover and explore food on their own, *without someone pushing it on them or praising them for eating.*

7. *Strive for stress-free mealtimes.* This isn't always easy with today's hectic schedules. "The hardest time for most families is dinner," notes Dr. Winchell. "Parents have all these expectations about how 'nice' families should behave at the dinner table. But in most households, by the time supper is served, everyone is so tired, hungry, and low on patience that the image of

perfection can never be reached. Battles erupt easily and frequently over the least little things."

Also, a lot of people think dinner is the best time for heated debates or discussions about schoolwork and other serious issues, notes Dr. Winchell. "But those subjects tend to generate a lot of stress, which has a negative effect on appetite," she says.

Also bad for the appetite are criticism and nagging, which most parents have a hard time resisting when they're sitting at the table, face-to-face with children who routinely spill milk, eat with their fingers, get food in their hair, never use a napkin, or talk with their mouths full.

It can help enormously if you set a few basic ground rules—for everyone at the table (including the adults) to follow:

1. No complaining about the food (if you don't like something, just push it to the side of your plate).
2. No criticizing (about what or how anyone else eats).
3. No trying to bribe or force anyone else to eat.
4. No fighting—about anything.

"Try to create a pleasant and unrushed environment," stresses Busch, "so your picky eater will look forward to family meals."

Is My Baby Too Thin?

Despite the fact that our culture tends to exalt thinness in adults, many people worry when they see a baby who doesn't have dimpled arms and pudgy cheeks. But most slender babies are just as healthy as their roly-poly peers.

"There's only so much you can do to influence how your baby grows," explains Dr. Barbara Kirschner. "Adult height and weight are basically preprogrammed at conception." Boys usually end up being a little taller than the midpoint between their parents' heights; girls, a little shorter. And the tendency to be thin, husky, or in between is linked to genes.

Of course, eating habits can affect a child's eventual size in either a positive or negative way. A malnourished child, for example, may end up being shorter than expected; a child who mainly eats junk food may end up overweight. Proper health care and exercise also play important roles in ensuring that a child meets his or her genetic potential.

So, if your baby is getting plenty of food but remains thin, and you, your spouse, or others in your immediate families have a tendency to be lean, small-boned or petite, there's probably nothing to worry about. As Dr. Kirschner points out, some babies from the time they're born have small appetites, while others seem to want to eat everything in sight. "As long as your child is following his own growth curve, there's no need to force your baby to eat more than he wants," she adds.

If thinness doesn't run in your families, but your baby is active, alert, generally content, and showing steady (even if it's slow) growth, there's still no need to worry. Children grow at different rates throughout their early years; while some are fast growers, others are late bloomers. In the end, most healthy children achieve the height and weight their genes prefer.

The time to be concerned—and to call the doctor—is

*when a baby under twelve months old fails to gain
weight, or loses weight, for two or more months in a
row.* This could signal either underfeeding or a medical
problem, such as an inability to absorb certain nutrients, an infection, or a chronic disease. In such cases,
prompt medical attention is essential.

"You should also be concerned if an older child
shows a sudden swerve off her growth or height
curve," notes Dr. Kirschner, "or her thinness is accompanied by anxiety or depression. Emotions can have a
big impact on a child's desire to eat."

2 PICKY TODDLERS AND PRESCHOOLERS

AGE FLAG: 1 TO 4 YEARS

A CHANGE IN APPETITE

Once your child is out of the milk stage and eating
most of his meals and snacks with the rest of the family, you can almost count on facing both food refusals
and finicky food preferences. You may even become
alarmed at how little your child seems to be eating and
how slowly he seems to be growing, compared to the
pace he set during his first year. "This is the age when
parents typically come into the office feeling all upset
because their child seems more interested in playing
with food than eating it," says Dr. Williams.

But it's perfectly normal for a child's appetite and
growth rate to slow down, he adds. During the first
year of life a baby's weight can easily triple, but in the

second year it tends to increase at a much more leisurely pace. From now until your child is five or six years old, you can expect him to put on a modest four or five pounds a year, and to go three or four months at a time without increasing his weight at all.

The logical result of this slower growth rate is a reduced need for calories and a smaller appetite.

Stronger Opinions

It's perfectly normal for children this age to show stronger likes and dislikes when it comes to different foods. Toddlers and preschoolers frequently:

• Insist on certain foods or eating rituals to help themselves feel more secure and confident about being the littlest members of a very big world. "You may think it's boring to eat the same thing every day," notes Felicia Busch, "but to a child who's trying to navigate her way through babysitters, day care, preschools, and so forth, it can actually feel reassuring to see that same old sandwich on the same old plate, with a familiar piece of fruit and a glass of milk nearby."

• Lose their appetite because of intense emotions (for example, they're having too much fun playing with their friends or learning a new skill; they're too excited about an upcoming party, too upset by conflicts between their parents, or too frightened by their own fantasies about monsters and bad guys).

• Reject foods (even old favorites) on the basis of how they look. "The sense of smell is not fully developed until a child is about four or five years old," explains Mary Abbott Hess. "However, the shape, color, and presentation of food are very important to children this young." Familiarity is also vital. "This is a time of intense reactions to anything different, uncertain, or new," says Marjorie Sutton. "It often takes fifteen or twenty exposures to a food before a child this age will feel brave enough to try it."

• Show huge swings in appetite. "It's not unusual for children this age to eat well for two or three days, and then eat very little the next day," says Dr. Williams. "But over the course of a week or so, most picky eaters who have access to healthy foods manage to consume a sufficient, balanced diet."

Act Natural

Although difficult, it is extremely important to take food refusals and finicky eating habits in stride as soon as they first appear. "Instead of worrying about how to get your child to eat, you should be concentrating on how *not* to react when picky eating occurs," notes James Windell.

Dr. Garber agrees. "Very often, a child's resistance to food is maintained by the pressure and attention she gets for *not* eating," he says. "So the best way to discourage picky eating is to act like you don't care."

If you panic and try forcing (or tricking) your child into eating, or into swallowing foods he finds distasteful, you'll only make matters worse. Even at the innocent age of one or two, a child who feels he's being forced to eat something will attempt to defend his rights. He may cry and throw a tantrum, for instance, or push the bowl off of his high chair in brazen defiance. He may even take a swipe at the spoon he sees heading toward his mouth. Eventually, instead of viewing mealtime as a pleasant experience, he'll see it as a prime time to test, tease, and terrorize you—and instead of eating more, he'll begin to eat less.

"Try to remember that your job is to provide a variety of healthy foods, and let your child choose what to put in his mouth," adds Felicia Busch. "If you show too much frustration or overinterest in what your child chooses, it will come back to haunt you tenfold as your child matures."

THIRTY WAYS TO ENCOURAGE EATING—WITHOUT FORCING, BRIBING, OR BEGGING

If you feel a strong need to *do more* (many concerned parents don't feel comfortable unless they're actively trying to "solve" their child's behavior "problems"), you can try some of the following behind-the-scenes strategies for shaping your child's diet. However, if you decide to use these, it's extremely important to keep your efforts and goals to yourself. If your child even suspects that you're trying to trick her into eating something she thinks she doesn't want, you'll be back to square one with a kid who won't eat, and daily fights over food.

Also, keep in mind that there's no single strategy that will work with every child or in every situation. To make sure you have lots of options, here are thirty of the best ideas offered by the pediatricians, nutritionists, child psychologists, and parents interviewed for this book.

1. If your child is an extremely picky eater, start each meal with the (wholesome) foods you know your

child likes; don't even offer her any of the foods you know she hates for a few months. Your goal is to get her to approach the dinner table with an anticipation of pleasure rather than dread. Once you notice that happening, very, very slowly add some eensy-weensy portions of new foods that she hasn't yet decided to despise. Then let her decide when to sample them.

2. If your child is still drinking from a bottle, find a way to wean her off it (reread the tips for weaning in Chapter Three). "After age two, a bottle is not appropriate, because it encourages overconsumption of milk and juice, which can kill the appetite for solids," says Dr. Ayoob. "Parents are often afraid to take the bottle away, because they think their picky eater will then consume nothing—but that never happens," Dr. Ayoob adds. "As soon as the bottle is gone, the child stops relying on liquids for most of her calories and starts eating more solid foods, and, it is hoped, a more balanced diet."

3. Expose your child to lots of different foods, even if you think he won't eat them. "When picky eaters see other people enjoying new foods, they often become intrigued," Mary Abbott Hess says. "A woman once came to my office feeling very upset because she was convinced her toddler would only eat pureed baby foods," she adds. "So I did an experiment. I put a bowl of gefilte fish balls within reaching distance of the child and continued to chat with the mother. While we were talking, the child grabbed and ate six of the fish balls. The mother was astonished because she never dreamed her child would want an 'adult' food like that."

Hess adds, "Never assume your child can't or won't

eat something without first offering her the chance to try it."

4. Never overwhelm your child with too many new foods at once. "Always offer something new alongside something you know she likes," advises Dr. Lilienfeld. "The more familiar food will help her feel less suspicious of the unfamiliar one."

Two good staples to have at every meal (because most children will eat them) are:

• Bread, which is a good source of fiber, iron, and B vitamins; and

• Milk, which is chockful of calcium.

"Most children like these foods," says Dr. Lilienfeld. "And if a kid eats nothing else, the parent can still rest easy knowing that their child consumed *something* nutritious."

5. Offer your child lots of opportunities to make her own food choices. For example, if she's hung up on white bread and cheese sandwiches, tell her she can have that at one meal each day. Then let her choose whether it will be at breakfast, lunch, or dinner. Or, tell her she can choose to have half the sandwich at lunch and half at dinner. Other possibilities:

— "Would you like your bread and cheese sandwich before you eat your apple, or after?"

— "The sandwich course comes after the vegetable course: So which would you prefer—carrots or broccoli?"

— "If you're still hungry after you finish your cereal, you can choose to have a sandwich or a piece of fruit. Let me know what you decide after you eat your cereal."

6. To encourage a more varied diet, ask your child

to list all the foods he likes. "Write them down on index cards," suggests Felicia Busch. Or cut out pictures of the foods he likes from newspaper flyers, magazines, or food boxes, and paste those on the cards. "Then put the cards in a hat and ask him to pull one out each day. Serve him whatever food is on the card during one of the day's meals." (But don't insist he eat it.) Another variation is to have him identify some new foods he'd like to try, and pull one of those out of the hat each day.

7. If your child has recently been potty trained, get in the habit of asking him to use the bathroom before meals. As Dr. Schwartzman points out, "A lot of times, young children will resist using the potty as long as they can, or they'll forget to use it because they're so busy playing. But then, when they sit down at the table, they can't eat because their bowels are making them uncomfortable."

8. Help your child work up an appetite. "Even the pickiest eater will eat when she's hungry," says Dr. Lilienfeld. "And the hungrier a child is, the more inclined she'll be to eat new foods and enjoy foods that are not her usual favorites." One way to increase hunger at meals is to readjust the snack schedule. For instance:

—Plan for no more than two snacks a day, and serve them only if your child requests them. "With extremely picky eaters," says Dr. Ayoob, "you may need to forego snacks for a while, so the child can build up an appetite."

—Offer a choice of nutritious foods during snack times, to fill in the nutritional gaps caused by eating poorly at scheduled meals, and to discourage your child from filling up on junk.

—Keep snack portions small, so they give a boost, but don't fill your child up.

9. Limit your child's intake of juice, soda pop, and other sweet drinks. "The first question I usually ask when a parent brings in a child who's a picky eater is, 'How much juice he is drinking?'" notes Dr. Merritt. "A lot of times I find out the child is getting 400 calories a day from juice drinks. No wonder he's not eating! I don't find much use for juice in the diet," adds Dr. Merritt. "All it does is fill a child up with empty calories."

Dr. Ayoob agrees. "Parents are usually happy when their picky eater drinks juice, because they think it's nutritious," he says. "But juice is not the nutrition bargain they imagine. I usually limit picky eaters to four to six ounces of juice (diluted with water) a day—and I strongly advise against letting a child carry around a bottle or cup of anything."

10. If your child is picky only when it comes to eating meals, but always wants dessert, don't refuse the dessert. Instead, start serving nutrient-rich foods for dessert. For example: low-fat yogurt with sprinkles on it, fresh-fruit kabobs, slices of fresh fruit with a yogurt dip, slices of cheese, whole-wheat toast sprinkled with cinnamon and sugar, baked apples, milkshakes made with yogurt and fresh fruit, etc. That way, if all she eats at a meal is dessert, you'll still know she got something nutritious into her system.

11. If the mere mention of a specific food makes your child want to choke, gag, or vomit, don't put it on her plate when the rest of the family eats it. "There's

no point in hassling your child over foods you know she hates," notes Dr. Winchell. "You can't convince her taste buds to change before they're ready."

Nor can you force a child not to gag. Some children have extremely sensitive throats and need extra time to get used to coarser food textures. With such children, a slow, relaxed approach to eating is essential.

12. Serve the foods your child thinks she hates in new ways. For example, my younger son refused to eat carrots until one day I decided to cut them in circles rather than long sticks. My older son claims to hate spaghetti, but if I serve him bow ties or shells, he practically vacuums them up. And neither of my children will touch a fresh banana, but if I prepare "hors d'oeuvres" (frozen banana slices topped with peanut butter and raisins) they fight over who gets more.

"Even adults respond differently when the same foods are served in new ways," notes Hess. "If I put out a bowl of oranges on a table in my office, the fruit will sit there untouched for days; but if I slice a few oranges into wedges and place them around the bowl, everyone who walks by will take one."

Anytime you can reduce a food into a bite-size finger-food format, you increase the chances that your child will eat it, she adds. Think in terms of hors d'oeuvres rather than entrees. "Children love foods that are small, colorful, crunchy, and interesting. And, since they're very tactile, they tend to favor foods they can eat with their hands."

13. If the food you're serving is somewhat dry and hard to chew, add a little juice or sauce to it. According to Mary Abbott Hess, children this young often prefer moist textures. "They have less saliva than older eaters,

so food that is dry and hard tends to get stuck in their mouths," she adds.

14. Make new foods more appealing by giving them fun or interesting names. "This works well with both of my sons," says mom Holly DeGregori. "One of their favorites is something I call 'Barney' soup, which is basically a tomato-based vegetable soup with blue food coloring added, to make it look purple. They love to help make it and eat it because of the *Barney* connection."

I've had similar success with this strategy. For instance, my older child always used to refuse rice, until one day I decided to mix it with some colorful bite-size vegetables and call it "Happy Rice." Now, he actually requests it (as in, "Mom, can we have Happy Rice tonight? *Please!*"). Be creative. Preschoolers have active imaginations and a great appreciation for word games. A new food name may tickle your child's mind and tummy.

15. Avoid serving foods that are either very hot or very cold. If your child burns his tongue on a food, he's going to be wary the next time he sees it. "In general," says Hess, "children prefer foods that are like Goldilock's porridge: not too hot and not too cold, but just right." That way, they can dig right in.

16. If you are seriously concerned about your finicky child never eating from a particular food group, find ways to use foods in that group to enrich the foods she will eat. For example, if she won't drink milk, you can still add milk to her diet by using it to mix her oatmeal or pudding or mash her potatoes; if she won't eat vegetables, you can grate them up and add them to her favorite entree; if she's short on fiber, you can add

apple slices to her pancakes or whole-wheat flour to her baked goods. And if you're really desperate and she won't eat fruit, you can slice up some strawberries and bananas and add them to a mound of whipped cream—with a cherry on top!

"With my first child, I became a master of disguise," says Carol Spelman. "I cut or finely chopped meat and vegetables (the foods she wouldn't eat) and mixed them into everything from spaghetti sauce to macaroni and cheese, grilled cheese sandwiches, and scrambled eggs (the foods she loved)."

More than anything, enriching foods will put *your* mind at rest. But don't go overboard on this, warn the experts. Your ultimate goal is still to raise a child who makes healthy choices on her own. If you're always hiding the good stuff, she's not going to learn that those foods are important ingredients in a healthy diet.

17. If your child is suspicious of *anything* new she sees on her plate, establish a "one-taste" rule. Explain that your child is not expected to eat everything you serve her, but before she can insist that she hates something, she must take at least one taste. She doesn't have to swallow the food if she doesn't like it—just touch it to her tongue.

Then, if she tastes the food and still hates it, comment briefly on how great it is that she's willing to try new foods before she decides to reject them. If she tastes it and wants more, acknowledge her bravery, but in a low-key way: "I'm so glad you tasted it and discovered you liked it. I'll be happy to give you a larger serving."

18. Don't try to convince your child to eat by lecturing her on the impact of diet or of different foods on

her health. And try to avoid telling her that certain foods are good, while others are bad. Children this age don't have much interest in health and can't really understand the concept of clogging one's arteries with food.

"You *can* teach a young child to start following the Food Guide Pyramid," notes Hess. "But you don't have to. If your child sees the rest of the family eating lots of grains, vegetables, and fruits, moderate amounts of meat and dairy products, and small amounts of fats and sweets, she's going to learn that that's the best way to eat."

Setting a good example also works best when it comes to encouraging an adventurous attitude toward food. "Studies show that cultural and social eating habits have more influence than individual taste preferences on a person's diet," Hess notes. "That's why you see toddlers in Mexico eating hot chilies, and preschoolers in East India enjoying curry. Children learn to like what their parents eat."

19. Every now and then, add something fun to the feeding routine. For instance, cut your child's food into a special shape or create a colorful design on her plate. One Halloween, for instance, I used pumpkin, witch, and cat cookie cutters to shape my son's sandwiches and cheese slices. Other parents have tried using colorful plastic spoons to brighten up a meal, special plates that the child has designed or that bears the child's name, or special paper napkins with the child's favorite cartoon characters.

But don't let your child manipulate you into making every plate of food into a funny face or every meal into a special event. (Save this tactic for your most desperate feeding moments!)

20. Get your child involved in meal preparations and routines. Even a two-year-old can help with:

- setting and clearing the table;
- ripping up lettuce leaves for salads;
- helping you pour ingredients into a mixing bowl and stirring the batter;
- picking out fruit and vegetables at the store; and
- making colorful name cards and other decorations for special meals.

"When a child feels she's made an investment in creating a meal, she's more likely to want to eat some of the food," says Marjorie Sutton.

Another similar option: encourage your child to play alongside you in the kitchen while you're cooking. Set up a mini kitchen, for instance, using old food boxes and cans as props, or buy some fake food for him to experiment with. While you're stirring and chopping and frying, he can be preparing a pretend meal. Later, spend time in his fantasy kitchen sampling all the interesting concoctions he comes up with. (Then maybe he'll be more open-minded when it comes to sampling yours!)

21. Take your child food shopping and let her touch and smell a variety of foods. Encourage her to pick out one or two things she's never tried before, and then work them into a family meal. Also, take her to local farms and orchards when various fruits and vegetables are in season, and let her pick her own supply of fresh foods.

As Sutton notes, "Often children are more adventurous about tasting new things when they're outside the home or involved in the food-gathering process."

22. Let your preschooler help with meal planning by selecting one of the foods to be served at supper each night. If it's something he can help prepare—all the better. Or have him look through supermarket flyers and cut out pictures of the foods he likes best. He can paste these onto a paper and carry it as his personal shopping list the next time you go to the grocery store. Finding the foods on his list will help keep him from nagging you for treats when you're in the store, too!

23. Look for children's books that encourage either healthy or adventurous eating, such as the classic Dr. Seuss volume *Green Eggs and Ham*. Read them with your child and talk about the characters, the story, and the foods involved.

24. Don't make food the focus of conversation either at the table, or when you're away from it. That doesn't mean you can't talk about your favorite foods sometimes, or discuss how much you enjoyed a new food or special meal. But don't get caught up in daily discussions about how much your child (or another family member) ate, what he ate, or how he ate it. And try not to comment when your child's eating habits either fulfill or fall short of your expectations.

In particular, you want to avoid phrases like:

- "You're hardly eating anything today."
- "You eat like a bird these days."
- "Why aren't you eating your vegetables?"
- "What's wrong? You ate those yesterday, but you won't even touch them today."

- "I'm so proud of you for eating all your supper."
- "I can't believe you're not eating—do you know how hard I worked to prepare something you'd like?"
- "If you finish up all your carrots, I'll take you to the store for ice cream."

"Good or bad, comments about eating tend to shift a child's focus away from eating because he's hungry, to eating because he wants to please—or displease—other people," notes Mary Abbott Hess.

25. If your child is recovering from an illness, don't be too eager to push food down her throat. If you force food before your child's natural appetite has returned, it may make her even more resistant to eating and prolong her recovery.

26. Look for ways to lessen the stress in your child's life. If there's a new baby in the family or a parent is ill, a child may express her anxiety or emotions by not eating. Rather than plead, coax, or beg your child to eat, work behind the scenes to lessen the stress, or help your child learn to handle her stress in healthier ways (for instance, by talking to a grown-up, drawing a picture, or kicking a ball around outside).

27. Make the most of breakfast. "This can be a wonderful meal for picky eaters," notes Corinne Montandon. "After sleeping for ten or so hours, they usually wake up feeling hungry enough to eat just about anything." Now's the time to fit in some of those trickier food groups, she adds. "You don't always have to serve cereal. You can offer a grilled-cheese sandwich, cheese and toast, yogurt and a slice of toast, even leftover pizza."

28. Make food jags work to your advantage. "For instance, if your child is hung up on peanut butter," says Felicia Busch, "find ways to work that ingredient into a varied diet." You could serve peanut butter on a bagel for breakfast; a turkey sandwich and a peanut butter cookie for lunch; and celery sticks spread with peanut butter at supper.

29. "Make sure your child sits down to eat," notes Dr. Lilienfeld. And turn the TV off. "Children are more likely to eat more if they're concentrating on food, rather than on toys or the TV," he adds.

30. Give your child time to change her finicky eating habits. Once a habit of picky eating has begun, it can take a long time to break. As you implement any of the strategies above, try to keep in mind that nothing's going to change overnight. Your child will need lots of time—and you'll need lots of patience—before significant changes will occur.

Your Distaste for a Food Can Influence Your Child's Reaction

When feeding a picky eater of any age, it's important to think about your own attitudes toward the foods you're serving. You may be influencing your child without even realizing it.

"One of my cousins came to me because her seven-month-old didn't like any vegetables, aside from corn and carrots," says Mary Abbott Hess. "I decided to put a mirror behind the child's high chair, so we could see my cousin's face as she fed the child. It turned out that when she was feeding the baby something she liked, she would smile. But when she fed the child beets and other vegetables she disliked, she usually made a sour face, as though she were saying, 'Isn't this awful?' It turned out the baby was responding to her nonverbal cues.

"I had another mother come in and tell me her child wouldn't drink milk because he had a milk allergy. I asked her whether the allergy had been medically confirmed and she said no. So I asked her how she knew about it, and she told me that every time her child drinks milk and she asks him, 'Do you feel sick yet?' he answers 'Yes.' Without even realizing it, she was teaching him to reject milk."

SETTING LIMITS ON PICKY EATING

Very often, parents get so worried that their picky eater isn't getting enough nutrition that they go overboard in fulfilling food requests. You should consider yourself guilty of this if you've ever:

- followed your child around the room with a spoon;
- allowed him to eat in places you normally consider inappropriate (such as in the car or in bed);
- cooked him a special meal just minutes after cleaning up the kitchen;
- allowed him to run back and forth from the table to his toys all during a meal; or
- let him have more sweets than you normally would, because those are the only foods he ever wants to eat.

But don't be too hard on yourself for trying. "Feeding a picky eater is tricky, especially if your child is

leaving out entire food groups from his daily menu,"
notes Dr. Ayoob. "You don't want to refuse your child
food when he tells you he's hungry."

On the other hand, you shouldn't allow a picky eater
to control your life with food requests, eat nothing but
junk food, or grow up thinking that he doesn't have to
follow the family's eating rules.

"There's a difference between denying a child food
and denying him an unbalanced diet," says Dr. Ayoob.
If food requests are unreasonable or largely unhealthy,
there's no reason not to set limits (as in, "If you're still
hungry, I'll be happy to rewarm your dinner, but there
are no seconds on ice cream").

"State your position, without getting angry or responding to your child's inevitable pleas," says Dr.
Ayoob. "The worst that'll happen if he doesn't eat anything is that he'll show up even hungrier—and probably eat something healthy—at the next scheduled
snack or meal."

IF EATING DOESN'T IMPROVE

If, despite your best efforts, your child's picky eating
continues, and you're worried that it's affecting her
health, there are two more important steps you should
take:

1. *Keep a food journal.* Your impression of how
much your child eats and her actual consumption may
not be as synchronized as you think. One of the best
ways to find out how well they match is to keep a journal of what your child eats for a week. "Write down

every bite your child takes," advises Dr. Garber. Also, be sure to record:

- the time of each meal or snack;
- what your child was doing or feeling when the food was offered;
- how much your child ate;
- where the food was eaten.

"This kind of diary can be a real eye-opener for a parent," notes Dr. Garber. You may discover that your child is actually eating more than you thought or better than you thought. Or, you may discover that there are certain food groups you're not consistently serving, or ways you could reschedule meals and snacks to make sure she comes to the table hungry.

In addition, a journal can help you recognize the kinds of associations you may be making with food (for example: Do you frequently offer cookies when your child comes to you for comfort? Do you use food as a focal point for family outings and activities?) as well as the associations your child may be making (Is she whining for snacks whenever she's bored? Does she try to eat to make others happy?).

Of course, a diary can also serve to confirm your fears, if your child really isn't eating enough for a person her age and size—which brings us to the next step:

2. *Take the food journal, and your child, to a pediatrician or registered dietitian if you still have doubts or concerns.* There is no substitute for professional advice when it comes to your child's health. A pediatrician can rule out any medical problems that may be causing your child's poor appetite, and a registered dietitian

can guide you in making any necessary changes in what or how you feed your child.

Does My Child Need Vitamins?

"Studies show that the vast majority of American children are not vitamin deficient," says Dr. Williams. "However, I sometimes recommend vitamins for an extremely picky eater. But I always caution the parents that vitamins are a supplement—not a replacement—for a healthy diet."

BREAKING THE TWO-MEAL ROUTINE

Should you or shouldn't you make a separate meal for your picky eater?

The experts go back and forth on this one, but the bottom line seems to be: if you don't mind doing it, go ahead. "When you give your child more than one choice, you empower him to say, 'I don't like this' or 'I want more of this,' " notes Dr. Winchell. "And you avoid the issue of forcing."

However, if you're feeling overwhelmed by your child's special orders, or you just don't have the time or patience to make two or three different meals each night, there's no reason not to set limits.

"It's important to offer a child choices," notes Dr. Schwartzman, "but it's also important to teach her about limits. If you always act like a short-order cook, your child will develop unrealistic expectations about what family dining is all about—and you'll feel even more upset if he still doesn't eat."

Another problem with cooking special meals for a finicky eater is that it doesn't encourage variety. If you're always serving him old favorites, he may never feel compelled to try new foods.

The middle road is best, says Felicia Busch. "Try to balance every meal with some foods you know your picky child will eat, and other foods the rest of the family likes. That way, he'll be exposed to new foods, but he'll never have to leave the table hungry."

3 PICKY BIG KIDS

AGE FLAG: 5 TO 6 YEARS

WHEN THE WORST IS OVER

Most children begin to grow out of quirky eating habits around the time they leave home for kindergarten. "If you've managed to develop a fairly relaxed style of parenting, your punishments are not too harsh, and your expectations about food and eating have been reasonable, your child should be developing some fairly healthy eating habits by now," says James Windell.

Louise Bates Ames, author of *Your Five-Year-Old: Sunny and Serene,* agrees. "Not all five-year-olds eat three 'good' meals a day," she says. "But with their interest in finishing things, their normal perseverance, and their wish to do what other people want them to, fives often manage to clean up their plates, even though it may seem to you as if it's taking forever."

Food preferences, however, may still remain rather marked, adds Dr. Ames. "Children this age tend to like plain, simple cooking, and may thus like best meat, potatoes, a raw vegetable, milk, and fruit. Gravies, casseroles, puddings, cooked root vegetables, or anything complicated, with a strong taste, may be refused." On the other hand, she adds, "when a five-year-old is at a restaurant or visiting, he will eat foods that he would normally refuse at home."

The same holds true for six-year-olds, according to James Windell. "They don't like to experiment with unfamiliar foods," he says. "Given a choice, they would probably be satisfied with a steady diet of hamburgers and french fries."

In addition, like younger children, five- and six-year-olds can easily get caught up in the excitement of things (a birthday party, a soccer game, a test at school) and forget to eat; or, they may try to rush through a meal so they can get back to an interesting video they were watching or play outside with their friends. (Try setting a timer for fifteen or twenty minutes, to discourage rushing.)

Keep Being Patient

If picky eating worsens in this stage of development, there may be an underlying problem such as illness, stress, or anxiety. In addition, if food battles have been common in your household for some time, finicky eating is not likely to abate now on its own.

Your best bet is to have your child examined by his doctor, and start following the advice offered in this chapter for toddlers and preschoolers. Above all, try to eliminate any pressure you're applying to get your child to eat.

If left alone, most picky eaters do grow up to be adults with fairly normal eating habits. I can vouch for that myself. When I was little, I was about as picky as they come, mainly because of my sensitivity to taste and odor. But my parents didn't make a big deal of it. They served me whatever everyone else was eating, and if I didn't eat anything, they left me alone.

It still took me a long time to enjoy certain foods. For instance, I couldn't bear to eat tomatoes or cooked onions until I was in my twenties, but now I love both of them. I also hated rice and beans, but now they're among my staples.

There are certain things I still can't eat, such as fish and mushrooms. The smell and texture of those foods just turn me off. But I have absolutely no problems sustaining a hearty appetite—or a healthy weight!

Your picky eater may never develop an eclectic palate, but with your support, she will probably learn to like everything she needs to survive.

✕ FIVE

Serious Concerns: Getting a Child to Eat Less Junk

"My greatest food challenge is trying to regulate what my four-year-old daughter, Beth, eats outside the home," says Karen Mann (not her real name). "I have nothing against an occasional treat. But I'm often amazed at the frequency with which she's offered junk. For instance, one of her babysitters used to give her huge handfuls of Oreos in the afternoon for a snack; and on play dates, other parents have handed her things like chocolate lollipops and Creamsicles right before she comes home for dinner. Then she doesn't want to eat dinner. Plus, she's started complaining about my more nutritious snacks."

"But I hesitate to say anything," adds Karen. "I don't want to alienate other parents by seeming holier-than-thou about nutrition; I don't want to be the unpopular mom who serves boring snacks; and I don't want Beth to feel like the odd kid out because she can't eat what the other children eat. I feel really stuck!"

So do many other parents. Even those of us with picky eaters are often appalled when we see our children wolfing down french fries, drooling over doughnuts, and cramming in candy. We fear such food isn't good for our children, and we worry that it'll make them sick, overweight, or hyperactive. And yet . . . we *still* have a hard time drawing the line on junk food.

It's partly because we know that junk (food that is high in calories, fat, sugar, and/or sodium, but low on vitamins, minerals, and fiber) tastes good and brings people pleasure. And we like to see our children smiling. As Felicia Busch notes, "One of the main reasons adults give children junk food is because they enjoy watching them eat it." In addition, these foods can be amazingly effective at getting kids to quiet down and behave (just ask my son's bus driver, who routinely hands out Tootsie-Roll Pops).

But there is so much junk food around these days, and it's become such a part of our daily lives (it's even in school cafeterias!) that it's hard not to agonize over when to say yes and when to say no. Most parents eventually feel so overwhelmed that they either *give up,* and try to totally ban what they feel are the worst junk foods from their kids' diets, or *give in,* and let their children consume whatever they please.

But neither tactic is good for a child's health or well-being.

----------- ✳ -----------

The Real Junk

One parent I know won't let her children eat candy, but she will let them drink Coke. Another parent won't buy his kids french fries, but he'll let them have hot dogs twice a week. A third parent thinks fruit juice is healthy, but milkshakes are deadly. . . .

The more you ask around, the more you realize that everyone has a different opinion on what is and isn't junk. Fortunately, most nutritionists say it's not *what* your child eats, but *how much* and *how often* that really count.

Rather than worry about junk foods, say the experts, you should worry about a junk diet—*a consistent intake of more than the recommended amounts* of calories, fat, saturated fat, cholesterol, sodium, and sugar (see Chapter Two). Splurging now and then is okay, they say, but splurging every day is not.

✳

WHY BANNING JUNK DOESN'T WORK

If you tell your child, "You can't have any candy; it's bad for your health," she's probably not going to say, "Okay, I won't eat candy because it's bad for me. Can I have some broccoli instead?"

It's more likely she'll think, "Candy tastes so good. Why can't I have it? Other kids get to eat it. I want it, too. In fact, I need it. I've got to find a way to get it!" She may also start thinking, "Besides, I'm not going to let any grown-up boss me around! I'll eat what I want."

"Any time you try to ban or restrict a food, you automatically make it seem more desirable," says Dr. Williams. "Your child then spends *more* time thinking about and wanting that food than she would have spent eating it if you had just given her a small amount and let the matter drop."

Registered dietitian Sanna James agrees. "One of the things that makes junk foods so attractive to kids is that parents often forbid them," she explains. "I remember when I was growing up, there was a girl in my class who was not allowed to eat any candy at home. So every day after school, she'd race to the store and spend whatever pocket money she had on candy. The rest of us liked candy, of course, and occasionally bought it, but she was obsessed with it."

Other Drawbacks

Banning has lots of other drawbacks, too. For one thing, the ingredients that most parents would like their kids to avoid are almost impossible to evade in our culture. Take sugar, for instance. It's added to an astonishing array of things we eat, including items we don't even think of as sweet (such as ketchup, mayonnaise, crackers, cereal, peanut butter, and cough syrup). So your child is going to consume refined sugar whether you want him to or not. And, since all humans are born with a preference for sweet flavors, your child's sweet tooth isn't going to disappear just because you won't let him eat candy on Valentine's Day or cake on his birthday.

Another problem is that high-calorie, high-fat snacks and fast foods are so ingrained in our culture that trying to avoid them completely takes more skill and effort than the average parent has to spare. As soon as you try, you end up spending most of your free time with your child saying things like: "No, honey. Those aren't good for you. Have some grapes instead," and "I don't care if Melinda's mother lets her eat those, I don't think they're healthy."

In the process, you separate your child from her peers. As Ellyn Satter points out in *How to Get Your Kid to Eat . . . But Not Too Much,* "Food is culture, it's part of knowing what's going on in the world and feeling like a part of it." Would you want to be the only person on the playground who'd never heard of Happy Meals or Reese's Pieces?

The Eventual Outcome

Perhaps the greatest drawback of banning certain foods is that it generates negative feelings about food. "There's always a danger in teaching your child that some foods are 'good' for her, and others are 'bad,' " explains Sanna James. "If your child one day discovers that she really likes eating one of the 'bad' foods, she's going to feel badly about herself for liking it. She may also feel frightened, because she's worried that it'll do something bad to her body. Another possibility is that whenever she gets the chance, she'll overeat the food, to satisfy her cravings and assert her will."

WHY YOU CAN'T GIVE UP, EITHER

This doesn't mean you should move in the opposite direction and become so totally relaxed about junk food that you let your child eat whatever he wants, whenever he pleases. When it comes to food, the "if you can't fight 'em, join 'em" approach doesn't help a child learn to manage food choices.

While the research shows that most children will,

over time, choose a balanced diet—that's only if they're offered *an ongoing array of healthful foods.* There is no evidence that most kids can be trusted to eat wisely when the choices frequently include cookies, snack cakes, brownies, ice cream, candy bars, soda, and other sugary treats, or such high-fat favorites as hot dogs, hamburgers, chicken nuggets, french fries, and potato chips. "At a certain point, when faced with such temptations, children stop listening to their appetite center and start obeying their taste buds," notes Mary Abbott Hess.

"Plus, there are some children—like my two-year-old daughter—who seem to be born with the desire to eat nothing but cupcakes, cookies, and ice cream at every meal," says Dr. Kathy Merritt. "With such children, you really have to be careful about exposure to junk food, or that's all they'll ever eat."

The Ill Effects

No one knows exactly *why* humans develop preferences for sugary, salty, and high-fat foods, but the fact is, we do. Even newborn babies will favor a sweetened bottle of water over an unsweetened one, and children are fast learners when it comes to acquiring the taste for salt and fat. Unfortunately, the more they eat foods that are loaded with those ingredients, the more they crave them. And the greater their consumption, the worse the effects on their health.

Although the connection between childhood diets and adult diseases is not yet clear, it is certain that children who eat a steady supply of high-calorie, high-fat, and sugary foods face a greater risk of:

1. *Poor nutrition.* If your child is filling up on candy, cookies, juice, and hot dogs all day, she's not going to have much room left over for sandwiches, string beans, and apples. But if she doesn't eat those vitamin-rich foods, she won't get her required supply of essential nutrients.

"This is the biggest risk with junk foods," notes Sanna James. "They end up replacing the more nutritious foods in a child's diet."

2. *Obesity.* Most of the foods that fall into the junk category are not only low in nutrients, they're high in calories. While active children need a good supply of calories to fuel their energy levels and growth, they don't need a steady oversupply. Their bodies, like ours, are designed to convert extra calories into fat. And, as most of us know too well, stored fat means excess weight.

The birth-to-age-six stage is *not* the time to be worrying about your child's weight or putting him on a diet. But you should be aware that childhood obesity is a major problem these days. Studies show that over the past two decades, the number of six- to twelve-year-old children who are obese (more than twenty percent over the ideal weight for their sex, height, and age) has risen by about fifty-four percent, and extreme obesity (being more than forty percent over ideal weight) has jumped an astonishing ninety-eight percent.

This is not all due to overeating junk foods. Obesity is associated with a variety of factors, including genetics, activity levels, and diet. But many experts suspect that diet has played a major hand in the recent, rapid rise of obese American children.

3. *Tooth decay.* This is probably the most well-

known result of overconsuming high-sugar foods. But candy isn't the only culprit. "Sweet foods that stick to the teeth cause the most problems, particularly if they are eaten between meals," says Extension specialist Carolyn Raab. "Bacteria in the mouth feed on the sugars that stick to the teeth and produce acid, which slowly dissolves the surface of the teeth."

In addition, the most common cause of severe tooth decay in childhood is walking around or falling asleep with a bottle of juice, punch, or milk in the mouth.

WHY THE MODERATE APPROACH IS BEST

As with most things in life, the solution to the junk food dilemma lies along the path of moderation. You can't eradicate all those delicious-but-not-nutritious foods, so you might as well accept the fact that they exist and teach your child how to enjoy them—within the context of a balanced diet.

One of the strongest arguments in favor of this approach is that no one food, or type of food, is inherently harmful for a child. As Ellyn Satter explains in her book *Child of Mine,* "Nutritionists are fond of saying, 'There are really no junk foods, only junk diets.' Translated, that means that there are really no good or bad foods, it all depends on the context."

Just take potato chips. As Satter points out, they're high in fat and calories and low on nutrients. If you add them to a diet that's already laden with foods like ice cream, candy bars, and soda pop, you can safely view them as junk. They won't improve your child's nutritional status, and they may dull her appetite for more nutritious foods.

But what if your child is a pretty healthy eater? What if she's met all her nutrient requirements for the day, but needs some extra calories to fuel her active life-style? In that case, a modest serving of potato chips might be a smart choice. As Satter explains, "If her diet is lacking only in calories, the chips would be better for her than something like carrots because the chips would give more calories."

In other words, potato chips aren't *always* bad for your child's diet. Neither is candy. It's true that candy is mostly sugar, and that sugar doesn't contain any vitamins, minerals, protein, or fiber (all it really contributes to the diet is calories). But if eaten *in moderation, and within the context of a balanced diet,* it doesn't appear to do children any particular harm. It will promote cavities, of course, if your child isn't diligent about brushing; and in some children it produces a temporary drowsiness. But the bulk of the research shows that sugar is not the cause of obesity, hyperactivity, or diabetes; nor does consuming a moderate amount pose any known risks to long-term health.

Limiting Fat

Fat, of course, is a more worrisome ingredient because of its link to heart disease, stroke, certain cancers, and other illnesses in adulthood. Whether or not you have a family history of any of these diseases, you should certainly watch your child's fat intake after age two. But you needn't be obsessive about it.

When it comes to feeding your child an occasional bag of Fritos, or treating him now and then at the local burger joint, dietary fat should not make or break your decision. For one thing, there is still no hard evidence that what a person eats in childhood causes illness and disease later on. In their book *What Should I Feed My Kids?* Ronald E. Kleinman, M.D., and Michael S. Jellinek, M.D., point out, "A child will not develop heart disease by eating saturated fat. An eating pattern that includes leaner, low-fat foods and continues over thirty or forty years may be able to slow the accumulation of fatty deposits in the blood vessels of some people— which is why the whole population ought to eat a diet that's a little bit leaner—but no single food even repeated in the diet is going to make a big difference."

In addition, even fast-food fare—the king of fat in our culture—has some redeeming nutritional qualities. As Dr. Schmitt notes, "Although most of the food offered by fast-food restaurants is heavy on fat, high in sodium, and low on fiber, it also contains something from each of the major food groups." A meal consisting of a hamburger (on a bun, with tomato and lettuce), french fries, and milk, for instance, provides protein, vegetables, a bread, and a dairy product.

Considering that children usually eat a balanced diet over the course of a few days (rather than a few meals), that's not so bad. Your child can benefit from the nutrients that are present in the fast food, and then balance out the fat, calorie, and sodium content of that meal by getting plenty of exercise and eating healthier foods at subsequent meals.

Frequency and Quantity

What you need to watch out for most are *frequency* and *quantity.* "If your child is eating three big candy bars a day, or burgers and fries four times a week, *then* you should worry about junk food," says Dr. Winchell. At that point, the excess fat, sugar, calories, and sodium, and the lack of fiber and other nutrients in those foods would affect her ability to consume a balanced diet. But if you're talking about an occasional family outing to buy ice cream, one small piece of candy after dinner each night, or a monthly visit to a fast-food palace, it needn't be a concern.

"In the long run, allowing some junk into your child's diet is likely to cause fewer problems than imposing an all-out war on one food or category of foods," adds James Windell. "If your child feels she can indulge her curiosity and cravings for sweet, salty, or high-fat foods now and then, she's less likely to become obsessed with them." She's also less likely to overeat when they're offered or to eat them in secret or out of spite. Most important, if she's already eating a mostly healthy diet (and brushing her teeth regularly), she's not likely to suffer any ill effects from an occasional splurge.

1 BABIES AND JUNK FOOD

AGE FLAG: BIRTH TO 12 MONTHS

THE IMPORTANCE OF AVOIDANCE

With a baby—and especially a newborn—you only need to know one strategy concerning junk food: don't serve it. (This is the one age when banning is appropriate.) Your baby doesn't need food filled with fat, sugar, and salt; he doesn't yet want it; and he won't miss it if he never gets it.

Obviously, unless you're thinking of turning your baby's formula into chocolate milk (which, of course, should *never* be done), junk food won't become an issue until solid foods are started, sometime between four and six months of age. At that point, you'll probably notice that your baby, like most others, has a budding sweet tooth. He may prefer applesauce over spinach, or peaches over meat, for instance. And you may feel tempted to serve him sweeter or sweetened foods just to get him to open wide and swallow.

Try to resist this temptation. "If your baby prefers naturally sweet fruits to cereal or vegetables, don't avoid cereals and vegetables altogether," notes Dr. Ayoob. "Rather, add unsweetened fruit to the other foods, and then gradually decrease the amount over time, until your baby is eating the cereal and vegetables by themselves. Otherwise, your baby may get used to eating only sweet foods, and that can throw a diet out of balance." (Also avoid honey. With infants under a year, it is associated with botulism.)

As your baby progresses from pureed foods to finger foods, it's worth it to go out of your way to offer him the least sugary versions of the things he loves: plain Cheerios instead of Frosted Cheerios, for example; all-fruit jam instead of regular jelly; or French toast with sliced fruit instead of syrup. The only thing extra sugar will add to his diet is calories; your baby will be much better off filling his tiny stomach with foods that provide both calories *and* nutrients.

Holding off on sweets will also benefit you, since your child can't whine for cookies and cake if he doesn't know what they are. "Eventually, *someone* (most likely a grandparent!) will offer your child a treat, and the honeymoon will be over," notes Dr. Sendelbach. "But there's no reason to rush things. Let your baby taste and enjoy foods in their natural state first."

Hands Off the Salt Shaker

Although they do like things sweet, babies aren't born with a preference for salt. In fact, their systems aren't all that proficient at processing it. So adding salt to a baby's food to make it taste better isn't necessary. Nor is it helpful. High-sodium foods can put a strain on a baby's immature kidneys. Plus, they give your child a head start on craving salty foods. (It doesn't take long to *learn* a preference for salt.)

Reduce the Juice

Most people don't think of fruit juice as a junk food. In fact, they tend to think of it as nutritious. That's probably why a USDA study recently found that preschoolers consume four times more noncitrus juices today than they did twenty years ago.

Most nutrition experts, however, are not pleased by the increase. They point out that because it's so sweet, juice can have the same dampening effect on the appetite as other forms of sugar. So once your child starts drinking juice, try to limit the amount she drinks each day, and be sure, at this stage, to dilute it (add two or three parts water to one part juice). "Don't be afraid to offer water between meals when your child is thirsty," says Dr. Williams.

✳

Food Labels: Your Best Defense

Never judge a food by its packaging or its ad slogans. If you really want to make healthy choices when buying food for your child, get in the habit of reading the Nutrition Facts labels that appear on nearly all packaged foods. These wonderful little rectangles provide a wealth of information about a food's nutritional value. You don't have to be a brain surgeon to understand them, and they can be very useful when deciding between one brand of food and another.

Among the most important bits of data to look at on a food label are:

* *The ingredients list.* Since these are listed by weight, you can quickly see how big a role sugar, fat, sodium, and additives play in the food by looking at the first three ingredients. Remember, however, that sugar and fat go by many different names (see Chapter Two).
* *The fat data.* By dividing the number of calories listed on the label by the number of calories from fat, you can figure out what percent of the food's overall calories are fat calories. The higher the percentage of fat, the more you should question the food's nutritional value (especially if it's over thirty percent).

    You can also find out how many grams of fat are found in each serving, and how many of those grams come from saturated fat, which is the one you most want to avoid.
* *The sugar, sodium, and cholesterol content.* Again, whenever possible, choose the foods with lower values in each of these categories.

✳

❋

Avoiding Junk at Day Care

Most parents don't think about food when they're checking out a new day care or preschool for their child—but they should, according to Felicia Busch. "Good nutrition in the early years is just as important to a child's health and development as a warm, caring, and stimulating atmosphere," she says.

When you visit a new day care, ask to see the daily menu and make sure:

* The written menu reflects what's actually being served;
* A wide variety of foods are being served (not just the same old standbys that most kids like), and children are allowed to make choices;
* The person who's designing the menus understands children and nutrition, and the menus follow the Food Guide Pyramid;
* The caregivers eat with the children, and eat what the children eat (as opposed to standing around drinking soda and gobbling down chips);
* Mealtimes are relaxed, and the children are not forced to finish foods they don't like, but can have seconds of foods they do;
* Food is not being used to bribe, punish, or comfort the children;
* Holidays and special celebrations are not centered around junk-food feasting;
* Caregivers have a system for letting parents know when problems over food arise, and work with the parents in solving them.

If you like a day care but you don't like its food policies, let the director know, advises Busch. "Many places are willing to accommodate special food requests," she says. "I was able to convince one place my son went to to switch from two-percent milk to whole milk for the children under age two; another day care allowed me to supply my own containers of low-fat milk for my son over age two."

2 LITTLE KIDS AND JUNK FOOD

AGE FLAG: 1 TO 4 YEARS

EXPECT THE ISSUE TO GROW

As you move through the toddler and preschool years, junk food is bound to become more of an issue. Your child will be increasingly aware of what other people (including you) are eating, and increasingly vocal about wanting to taste foods you may not want him to have. Plus, if he's leaving the house to go to day care or preschool or just to play on a public playground, he's going to be exposed to a lot of delicious-looking things you don't stock at home—and he may become curious to try them.

Unfortunately, he'll also become more aware of advertising. "To hook kids on their brands, food and beverage marketers are using an increasingly broad array of devices," notes Michael F. Jacobson, Ph.D., executive director for the Center for Science in the Public Interest, in his book *What Are We Feeding Our Kids?*

(coauthored by Bruce Maxwell). These include everything from kids' clubs at fast-food restaurants to tie-ins with popular movies or TV shows; product placements in movies; premiums, toys, and clothes tied to a brand-name food; and dazzling TV commercials.

One of the biggest problems with these devices, says Dr. Jacobson, is that they distract children from the food itself. "Kids learn to choose a food because they like the characters that promote it or the prize inside, instead of because the food itself is good," he explains. "And to make matters worse, tie-in foods are often the least healthful foods on the market."

Standing Your Ground

Even so, this is not the time to start enforcing strict rules about junk food or telling your child that he can't have certain foods because they're bad for his health. For one thing, most children could care less about their health or what's good for them. They simply don't have the cognitive ability to understand a statement like, "You'd better go easy on the burgers and fries, or you may end up with clogged arteries when you're fifty." Toddlers and preschoolers operate on a much more primitive level, as in: "This tastes good . . . I want more." If you want to make a positive impact, you have to meet them on that level.

Another problem is that frequently saying no is a dangerous game with kids this age. Toddlers and pre-schoolers are preprogrammed to fight for their independence, and often do things (or whine) just because their parents said no. The more inflexible you seem about food requests, the more your child will fight to get his way, as in:

HIM: I want some chocolate graham crackers.

YOU: I'm not going to buy those; they have too much fat in them. Let's get the regular graham crackers instead.

HIM: I want the chocolate ones.

YOU: You can't have them, they're bad for your health. Besides, you liked the regular ones last week.

HIM: I want the chocolate ones. That's what Daniel eats. You have to buy them.

YOU: No!

HIM: Waahhh!

In this kind of exchange, no one wins. And as Sanna James points out, "If you battle over food choices, you set the stage for the kinds of bad eating habits that lead to eating disorders and weight problems in later life."

Holly Hughes, a mother of three, agrees. "I'm more concerned about making sure my children avoid unhealthy *thoughts* about food than unhealthy food because that's what does damage in the long run," she says.

The Subtle Strategy

A better approach is to work behind the scenes at reducing your child's exposure to junk food, and limiting his opportunities to eat it. Here's how:

1. *Practice what you preach.* We all have our weaknesses. For some, willpower falters at the sight of a chocolate-chip cookie or a chewy fudge brownie; for others, it takes a big bag of salty potato chips, a pint of rich, creamy ice cream, or a thick, juicy hamburger with lots of mayonnaise, ketchup, and onions.

What's your weakness?

Being aware of your own cravings for low-nutrition foods is important, because how you indulge yourself will have an impact on your child's future eating habits. No matter how conscientiously you guard your youngster's plate against stray grams of sugar, fat, and sodium, if you load up your own with fried food, salty snacks, or rich desserts, she's eventually going to notice the discrepancy and demand to eat like you do.

"It's very difficult for a child to see a parent enjoying candy or soda or chips and then hear that same person say, 'Don't eat that,' " notes Dr. Ayoob. "You have to think seriously about the kind of food habits you're modeling."

"Children do as their parents do, not as they say," adds Felicia Busch. "There is no way you can teach your child about good eating habits if you don't iron out the problem areas in your own diet."

2. *Don't bring junk food home.* If you don't think your child should be drinking four cans of orange soda every day, or eating a Snickers bar after every meal, and you're sick of fighting over when he can and can't have these foods, don't buy them anymore.

This simple strategy will not only limit the amount of junk your child consumes, it will discourage him from constantly begging for foods you'd rather he didn't eat.

Most nutritionists are passionate on this point. "A lot of times with food, parents forget that they're the ones in charge," says Busch. "I had one woman come to my office with a three-and-a-half-year-old son who would only drink Hawaiian Punch. The child was putting away two sixty-four-ounce bottles of it a day. The mother was upset and wanted to know what to do. But when I told her to just stop buying Hawaiian Punch, she looked at me like I had slapped her in the face. She thought the whole thing was the kid's problem, not hers."

Mary Abbott Hess has a similar story: "Once a parent came to my office and said, 'All my child will eat is cookies.' My reply was: 'Your child must be very advanced to be able to go to the store and buy all those cookies!' Some parents are far too timid about standing up to unreasonable food requests."

Sure, it's hard to say no. But in the long run, it leads to fewer food battles, Hess adds. Even the most skilled pint-sized negotiator can't argue for long if you lead him over to the cupboard and explain in a calm, matter-of-fact voice, "I'm sorry, but I can't give you a powdered doughnut right now because we don't have any in the house." It may not stop your child from crying or throwing a tantrum, but it will prevent a huge, drawn-out power struggle. As soon as your child realizes his battle is not against you, but against an empty cupboard, he'll give up the fight and find something more interesting to do.

Other Advantages

There's another big advantage to not buying the foods that you'd prefer your child not eat: you can say yes more often. If the only snacks in the house are foods that you approve of, you can respond to all food requests with a pleasant smile and a positive comment, such as, "Of course you can have some yogurt—I'll get it out of the fridge for you," or "Pick whatever crackers you'd like to go with your apple juice." It's the easiest way to take the power out of struggles over food.

Plus, it discourages children from whining for snacks when they're not really hungry. Ever notice how the sight of a cookie or a bag of chips can suddenly make you feel hungry, while the sight of a salad reminds you that you're full? When it comes to food, there's a big difference between hunger and desire—and children are just as susceptible to desire as adults are.

"I've noticed that if I buy a huge box of Fruit Roll-Ups at Sam's Warehouse, to save money, my kids' desire for them grows," says Cathy Gilfether, a mother of three. "They end up eating more than they normally would if I had just bought a regular-size box."

3. *Try to say yes to special requests.* While it's important to limit your child's exposure to junk foods, there's no point in making him feel deprived. So when requests for sweets and treats come in, don't respond with an automatic no. Instead, try to think of a reasonable way to let your child have what he wants without spoiling his overall diet.

Surprisingly, there are a number of ways to keep both of you happy. You could:

• *Buy miniature or bite-size versions* of your child's favorite treats. Most kids this age would be so thrilled to get *two* miniature candy bars, that it wouldn't occur to them that one regular-size bar would have delivered more actual candy (not to mention more sugar and fat!).

• *Buy the lowest-fat or least sugary/salty version* of the food your child craves. If he wants cookies, get him the low-fat ones; if he wants hot dogs, get him the kind made with turkey rather than beef; if he wants ice cream, buy him fruit-juice pops or sherbert; and if he wants pretzels, get him the brand with less salt. There are so many reduced fat/sugar/salt versions of popular foods on store shelves these days that finding alternatives shouldn't be too difficult. And, at this age, most kids won't complain that there's a difference in taste.

• *Bake your own version* of what your child requests, and use a recipe that's low in fat, sugar, and sodium. Or, bake miniature cookies, cupcakes, and other treats she loves.

• *Include a small amount* of the desired food in a homemade snack mix. I can usually satisfy my three-year-old's midafternoon cookie craving by putting three or four miniature cookies into a bowl full of healthier choices, such as low-fat crackers, raisins, and Kix. Sometimes, if he's in a real "chocolate" mood, I'll throw in a few chocolate chips. Then he's happy, because he thinks he's getting a big bowl of treats, and I'm happy because I know he isn't.

This strategy also works well with breakfast cereal. Rather than refuse to buy your child a box of cereal because its main ingredient is sugar, you can tell him you'll buy it if he agrees to mix it with a less sugary cereal. You can even let him choose which of the low-sugar cereals you approve of to put in the mixture.

Then, at home, give him a big bowl and some measuring cups, and let him go at it. Ask him to name his fabulous new concoction. Kids this age love to eat what they create.

• *Allow the less nutritious food,* as long as it's accompanied by more nutritious side dishes. For example, bring along an apple or some carrot sticks for your child to eat with a fast-food meal, or serve her milk with her cookies. "Whenever you're serving junk food, try to make it part of a nutritional package that for the most part is healthy," stresses Mary Abbott Hess. That way, you won't have to worry about your child's nutrition or feel compelled to remind her that what she's eating is bad for her health.

• *Limit the quantity.* If your child constantly whines in the grocery store for foods you don't feel are nutritious enough, tell him he can make one completely uncensored choice each time you shop. Then, no matter how awful his choice seems, agree to live with it. (You may even be surprised one day when he picks out a new kind of fruit instead of a new kind of snack.)

If he's constantly thinking about dessert during family meals, tell him ahead of time that each person gets one piece of pie (or cookie or slice of cake, etc.) with that meal, and he can have his whenever he wants. That way, he can decide whether to save it for last or eat it first. If he eats it right away and asks for more, you can simply say, "Sorry, only one piece per person tonight. But there's still plenty of chicken, string beans, and mashed potatoes if you're still hungry."

If he is, he'll eat; if he isn't, he'll eat more of the main course at the next scheduled meal.

• *Limit the frequency.* For instance, if your child

loves eating at Burger King, Pizza Hut, or Kentucky Fried Chicken, take out a calendar and let him pick one or two nights in the month when the family will go. If he's constantly begging for candy, tell him he can have one piece of candy per day, and that he gets to choose at which meal to enjoy it. If he's crazy about ice cream cones or tacos, let him pick one night a week to eat that food.

"You don't have to give in to every single food request your child makes," notes James Windell. "Sometimes, you will just have to say no." But if you usually offer a reasonable alternative, your no will end up sounding more like a yes, and your child won't walk away feeling angry and resentful (or hungry).

And it won't hurt if every now and then, you serve sweets or other treats when your child doesn't expect them. You don't have to do it big. Little things like using a gumdrop to crown a bowl of fruit, or putting miniature M&Ms in a snack mix help your child appreciate that he can enjoy all foods, but in different quantities.

✻

What's the Best Way to Teach a Young Child about Healthy Eating?

For many parents, that's the million-dollar food question. But the answer many nutritionists give is somewhat surprising: don't.

"In the toddler and preschool years, children shouldn't be learning about 'good' foods and 'bad' foods," stresses Felicia Busch. "They should simply be learning that food is something they eat when they're hungry, and don't eat when they're not."

That doesn't mean you can't occasionally say things like, "Milk helps your bones grow," or "Eating spinach will help you get big and strong like Popeye." According to Busch, "A little of that is fine. But don't do it at every meal, or every day. Kids this age should eat because they enjoy food, not because something is 'good' for them."

Sanna James agrees. "Children learn more from the example you set than from the words you speak," she adds. "If nutritious food is part of your child's daily life, and individual foods aren't demonized or idealized in your household, she'll eventually internalize the concepts of a healthy diet."

But what if your child is hungry and wants to eat brownies instead of broccoli? How do you promote one without villainizing the other?

"First of all, let your child have access to both," advises James. "Then, if she wants to know why she can have an unlimited amount of broccoli but only one serving of brownie, explain to her that the broccoli is an *anytime* food that people can enjoy anytime they want; brownies are a *sometimes* food that our bodies enjoy, but in smaller amounts." That way, she won't end up focusing so much on each food's *value* (or the notion that one is 'good' and the other is 'bad'), adds James.

If she presses you further with a "But *why*, Mommy?" question, you can always reply, "That's just the interesting way our bodies work, honey. Now, how about more broccoli?"

❋

4. *Avoid using junk food to reward, comfort, or punish.* This is a tough one. It means you shouldn't do things like:

- Give your child a cookie if she cuts her leg;
- Take her to Dairy Queen if her soccer team wins or she doesn't throw a tantrum in the grocery store;
- Tell her, "That's it. No dessert!" if she hits her sister during supper; or
- Promise a treat if she finishes her meal.

Despite the fact that foods that are high in fat, sugar, sodium, and calories are often extremely effective in these situations, using any type of food to soothe, reward, motivate, or punish a child leads to bad eating habits. "You needn't be extreme about this," says Dr. Garber. "If you give your child a few M&Ms as an incentive during potty training, it's not going to turn her into a candy addict."

But if you *frequently* give sweets and treats to reward good work, good behavior, or even good eating habits; you *only* give treats when your child has done something great or behaved properly; or you *often* withhold sweets and other foods to punish misbehavior, you'll turn eating into an emotional issue. "And then you'll get into all sorts of problems with your child wanting and whining for sweets, hoarding and overeating junk foods, and so forth," Dr. Garber adds.

5. *Be Smart about Snacks.* Studies show that young children get as much as a third of their total calories from snacks. That's a sizeable percentage—and a strong argument for making sure that your child's snack calories are accompanied by lots of other nutrients.

One good way to ensure this is to reserve any sweets or treats you serve for regularly scheduled meals, so your child won't build an association between snacking and junk food. Instead, when he's hungry for a snack, encourage him to sit down at the table (not in front of the TV) and eat foods that are rich in vitamins, minerals, and fiber, such as fruit and vegetable chunks with a yogurt dip, or low-salt pretzels. Unless your child's taste buds have already been spoiled by a diet of too much sugar, salt, and fat, he's not going to complain about the high quality of the food you serve—he's going to eat it.

What do you do if he does whine for cookies, chips, or other foods you feel are junk? Or if he starts complaining because his best friend's mother feeds him Pop Tarts and soda pop during play dates?

Don't give a lecture on the benefits of healthy snacks or remind him that your concern for his health proves that you're the better parent. Instead, try one of the following no-fight strategies:

• *Stand firm and say in a matter-of-fact tone,* "I'm sorry, but all we have for snack today is pear slices and cheese chunks. If you aren't hungry, we can clean up and go play." This is especially effective if you think your child isn't really hungry, because it gives him an easy way out ("Okay, let's go play"). But to make it work, you've got to remain calm and resist getting sucked into a debate. If he starts trying to convince you you're wrong, just say, "I guess that means you're not hungry. Let's clean up and go play."

• *Defuse your child's emotions* (before he reaches the tantrum stage) by giving him a small serving of the food he wants *along with* milk or some other healthier foods. For example, if he's three years old, you could make a game of it and give him three potato chips, three chunks of cheese, and three slices of pear. This works best when you know your child usually eats fairly well, and he's asking for a food that you find only marginally offensive.

• *Offer a choice:* "You can have chips today, but only at one meal. Would you rather have them now or at lunch?" Again, as long as he's not eating junk all day, there's no reason not to be flexible.

Plan Ahead

There's one other snack strategy every parent should remember: be prepared. Children have an uncanny ability to become hungry as soon as you're out of reach of your usual food stock—and often when you're in public. Without a moment's notice, they start getting cranky and demanding, and you feel enormous pressure to buy whatever kind of sweet or treat (soda, candy, chips, ice cream, nachos, etc.) is within easy reach. (Nutritious foods never are.)

The solution is to get in the habit of putting together a healthy snack pack *whenever* you leave the house with a child in tow. That way, there will always be something healthy on hand. Plus, it may discourage whining; once your child realizes that he can't use guilt to make you buy him something from the vending machine, he won't ask for food unless he really needs it.

6. *Limit TV Time.* There are two good reasons for this. One is that the less TV your child watches, the less exposure he'll get to all those persuasive television ads that promote low-nutrition foods. Studies show not only that the average child is exposed to more than 30,000 commercials a year, but that the majority of

food commercials aired during children's programs promote foods that are high in sugar, fat, or salt (such as candy bars, salty canned foods, fast foods, and chips).

Other studies show that the more commercial television preschoolers watch, the more they request specific foods—and specific brands—when shopping with their parents. "Experts have consistently found that the children who watch the most TV have the worst diets and the lowest levels of nutritional knowledge," notes Dr. Jacobson.

"It is so important to help your child decode food commercials," says Extension and nutrition specialist Ann A. Hertzler. "Most young children can't tell the difference between a commercial and a TV program," she adds. "It's up to you to explain that just because a cartoon character is on a package, it doesn't mean the food is better or tastier or more nutritious. Or just because a food is advertised on TV, it doesn't mean it should be eaten every day."

The second argument against too much TV watching has to do with exercise. "The average child watches about four hours of television a day," says Hertzler. Plus, children today watch videos and play video and computer games. "Those hours represent time that they're not playing outdoors, burning off excess calories," she adds.

7. *Relax about what your child eats away from home.* If you follow all of the other steps outlined in this section, this last one should be easy. "Your child eats about twenty-eight meals in a week," notes Mary Abbott Hess. "If most of those feature healthy foods, then you don't really need to worry if three or four

include junk, or he occasionally eats low-nutrition snacks when he's playing at a friend's house. His overall diet will remain balanced, and he'll learn that even treats can play a role in a healthy diet."

Of course, if there are certain adults whom you feel go way overboard in providing your child with nonnutritious snacks, you shouldn't hesitate to speak up. (I once had to ask my child's teacher to stop giving candy as a reward for good work!) And if all else fails, you can send your child out of the house with his own personal snack pack. But don't go that far if you don't have to. It never helps to make a child feel different from his peers.

IS MY CHILD TOO FAT?

Parents tend to get most upset about junk foods when they're also concerned about their child's weight. There's no doubt that consuming too much junk can lead to weight problems, even in early childhood. And with the rate of childhood obesity at an all-time high, it's an important concern.

However, it's also important to understand that children under age six should *not be put on a diet*.

"There is no absolute when it comes to children and weight," stresses Dr. Williams. "Many children go through stages when they are a little chunkier than usual," he explains. "But it's often just a normal result of the growing process, and they even out later on."

If There Is a Problem

The best thing to do if you suspect your child is overweight, or heading in that direction, is to call your pediatrician. With a young child especially, you can't always tell just by looking whether he's overweight. Lots of children go through plump stages; plus, many children whose parents are large-boned or big are naturally taller and heavier than their peers from the moment of birth. It's only by looking at your child's personal growth chart, and comparing his numbers to the typical body size of other family members, that a doctor can verify that a weight problem actually exists.

Even if there is a problem, don't panic—and still don't put your child on a diet! As Dr. Williams notes, "A diet that's not monitored by a pediatrician, a dietitian, or a therapist who specializes in pediatric weight management could be dangerous to your child's health."

In addition, if you start focusing too much on counting calories and fat grams, or start denying your child foods because they're too fattening, you open the door to more serious problems, such as battles over food, overeating of forbidden foods, and feelings of low self-esteem and resentment.

"Even when I see five-year-olds who weigh a hundred pounds, or six-year-olds who weigh 140, I don't start talking about diets," says Dr. Williams. "Instead, I tell the parents that we need to sit down and talk about ways to improve the entire family's way of eating. We look at things like how to cut down on junk food consumption, what kinds of snacks are most appropriate, how to help the child resist temptation, and how to add more physical activity to the daily routine. The goal is to help the child *gradually* lose weight, or maintain weight as he grows taller, by adopting the kinds of eating and exercise habits that will keep him healthy for the rest of his life."

The key to success, he adds, is getting everyone in the family involved.

---- ✳ ----

Supermarket Strategies

"The hardest time to resist a child's pleas for junk food is when you're grocery shopping," says Corinne Montandon. That's when all the forces of advertising and food-packaging combine to stimulate desire. To keep the whining to a dull roar:

◆ Avoid food shopping with your child when you're feeling tired, hungry, or stressed out. That's when your ability to calmly say, "Sorry, we're not buying that today. But you can choose between this or this" is bound to be at an all-time low.
◆ Never shop when your child is hungry; a rumbling stomach will only strengthen his conviction that he really deserves that bag of lollipops.
◆ Just in case he gets hungry from looking at all that food, pack a snack he can munch on while in the cart.
◆ Bring a special book or toy to distract him while you pick out the boring foods.
◆ If your child is capable of getting nonbreakable food items off the shelves and putting them in the cart, ask him to help you out. Give him a picture list of things to find.
◆ Talk before you shop about how you'll handle an in-store tantrum, if that's a chronic problem for your child.

---- ✳ ----

3 BIG KIDS AND JUNK FOOD

AGE FLAG: 4 TO 6 YEARS

KEEP WALKING THAT FINE LINE

The bad news is, as your children get older, it's going to get harder and harder to limit their exposure to junk food. "By the time they're five or six, most children are watching a lot more television and paying more attention to advertising and licensed character tie-ins to various foods," says James Windell. "They're also away from home more often, they're more likely to trade food during school lunches, and they're more eager to eat whatever they see other children eating." But they aren't any better at making the connection between what they eat and how their bodies function.

What's a parent to do? "Learn to live with it," he says. "To a certain degree, you've got to accept the fact that your child is going to be eating things you don't approve of when he's out of your direct sight," he adds. "But all that means is that you should be even more careful about serving nutritious meals and setting a good example at home."

There are two other steps you can add at this point:

1. *Encourage independence at snack time.* Five- and six-year-olds are more grown-up and capable, and more eager to show off their new skills. "This is a good age to start encouraging your child to practice making his own snack choices," notes Sanna James.

You should still buy only the foods that you approve of, but let your child decide what to eat, prepare the snack, and clean it up. Of course, it won't hurt if you try to make the foods you'd most like your child to eat accessible and attractive.

"Most children don't think ahead," says Sanna James. "They play and play until they get hungry, then they run to the kitchen and grab the first thing they see. The quicker you can get their attention with a nutritious food, the more likely it is they'll eat it."

For instance, she says, you can:

- Make vegetables more appealing by washing them, peeling them, cutting them into bite-size pieces, and storing them at eye level in the refrigerator in sandwich-size plastic bags; put salsa, bean dip, low-fat salad dressing, or yogurt into small, easy-to-open containers, so your child can use them as vegetable dips.
- Make fruit more tempting by washing it and then putting it out in a heavy traffic area; slicing it into "pick-me-up" pieces and storing them in small plastic bags in the fridge; or cutting it into bite-size pieces and freezing them, for hot-weather relief.
- Steer your child in a healthy direction by putting raisins and crackers in front of the cookies in your snack cupboard, or leaving a bowl of fresh-popped popcorn out on the table.

2. *Talk more about nutrition issues.* As your child's reading skills and awareness of the world grow, start talking about the Food Guide Pyramid and some of the basics of good nutrition. "A good way to start," says James Windell, "is to hang up a picture of the Food

Guide Pyramid and talk about how to read food labels."

Then, when you're in a store, trying to decide between two different types of cookies or cereals, you could ask your child to look at each one's Nutrition Facts label and tell you which kind has the least fat, sodium, or sugar. You could also talk about how the pictures and even some of the words on food packages can be deceptive.

You can even make a game out of it by challenging your child to find a cereal with six grams or less of sugar, or a cookie brand with less than ten percent of calories from saturated fat.

"You needn't make reading food labels or talking about nutrition the center of your world, or the main topic of conversation when you're with your child in a food store," adds Windell. "Just bring it up now and then. If your child acts bored or appears to be not listening, you're probably talking about it too much."

As with younger children, the example you set through the meals you serve and the snacks you eat will have a greater impact on your child's notion of healthy eating than any discussions the two of you enjoy.

So above all, be patient. You won't see the payoff for setting a good example until your child is much older and buying groceries and snacks on his own.

———————————————— ✳ ————————————————

School Lunch Solutions

Don't assume that lunches at your child's school are healthy just because they're being served at school.

More than a few cafeterias rely on hot dogs, hamburgers, french fries, nachos, ice cream, and other foods that are high in fat and sugar. And thousands more sell brand-name fast-food products, such as pizza from Pizza Hut and tacos from Taco Bell.

If your child's school lunch menu doesn't reflect the guidelines of the Food Pyramid, it's worth it to speak to the director of food services and request healthier foods. "You should also help your child decide ahead of time what he'll choose when he's in the lunch line," says Corinne Montandon. "It's hard for children to make good decisions on the spot with lots of other kids around. If there's something on the menu he hates, pack a lunch for that day."

With kids who brown bag it, don't expect everything you pack to be eaten. Your child may only eat a few bites, trade one item for another of lower nutritional value, or not eat anything at all. A good way to make sure your child eats most of what he brings is to have him help you make the lunch the night before. "Give him some reasonable choices, but let him decide on, prepare, and wrap the foods himself," says Montandon.

"Also, have your child bring home whatever he doesn't eat, so you can get a feel for what not to pack, and which food groups to encourage at snack time," she adds.

*

Final Thoughts

A leap of faith. That may be what you'll need to take to follow some of the advice in this book. Not because the advice itself is in any way radical or daring or dangerous. But because it requires a new way of thinking about food and feeding.

To make it work—to become truly relaxed about your child's eating—you'll have to let go of a lot of the myths our generation of parents grew up with. For instance:

- The idea that "cleaning" one's plate is more important than ending a meal when your body tells you it's full;
- The notion that "meat and potatoes" are the ultimate symbols of good nutrition, and that "three squares a day" are what keep a child healthy;
- The feeling that as a parent you are somehow responsible for making your child "eat right," even when he claims he isn't hungry;

235

- The hope that if you give your child lots of food or lots of treats, she'll know just how much you love her.

You'll also have to trade in all those safe-sounding rules about "eating vegetables before you can get dessert" and "taking at least three bites of any new food on your plate" for the three rules that are so simple and logical, it's hard to believe they'll work:

1. Eat when you feel hungry.
2. Eat a variety of foods from each of the major food groups.
3. Stop eating when you're full.

But Go Ahead: Take the Leap

I guarantee that leap of faith will land you in a better place when it comes to feeding your child.

I know—I've been working on breaking a lot of bad feeding habits myself as I've written this book, and it hasn't been easy. Those old myths and notions die hard, even when you understand that they no longer make nutritional sense.

But the amazing thing is, the less I worry and nag about what my kids eat, the better they actually eat.

The other night, I witnessed a minor miracle at my own dinner table. The New York Yankees had just won the game that got them into the 1996 World Series, and my husband and my older son Gus were so excited that we spent the entire meal talking about baseball (instead of noticing what and how the kids were eating). Every now and then, Teddy (the picky eater) would come up with a question like, "Mom, what are 'ankees'?" or "Dad, did the 'ankees' win?" But for the most part, he sat at his end of the table, and quietly ate—and ate and ate!

By the end of the dinner, Teddy had put away three helpings of macaroni and cheese, a piece of bread, and five raw carrots—without anyone once having said anything even remotely like, "How about another bite?" or "Try these carrots—they're yummy!" And, even more amazing, Gus didn't ask three million times what we were having for dessert and when he could have it.

Plus, we actually had a conversation—instead of a correction-fest—at the dinner table.

My conclusion: Either the Yankees have to win a lot more World Series, or I just have to keep remembering that when it comes to children and eating, the less said, the better.

Just give them a good variety of food, and they'll eat what they need to stay healthy.

Resources

BOOKS

Ames, Louise Bates, Ph.D., and Ilg, Frances L., M.D. *Your Five-Year-Old* and *Your Six-Year-Old*. Dell, 1981

Barness, Lewis A., M.D., Editor. *Pediatric Nutrition Handbook*, 3rd Edition. American Academy of Pediatrics, Committee on Nutrition, 1993

Coyle, Rena, and Messing, Patricia. *Baby Let's Eat!* Workman Publishing, 1987

Eisenberg, Arlene, Murkoff, Heidi E., and Hathaway, Sandee E., B.S.N. *What to Expect the First Year*. Workman Publishing, 1989

Forehand, Rex, Ph.D., and Long, Nicholas, Ph.D. *Parenting the Strong-Willed Child*. Contemporary Books, 1996

Galinsky, Ellen, and David, Judy. *The Preschool Years*. Ballantine Books, 1988

Garber, Stephen W., Ph.D., Garber, Marianne Daniels, Ph.D., and Spizman, Robyn Freedman. *Good Behavior*. St. Martins Paperbacks, 1991

Gershoff, Stanley, Ph.D., Whitney, Catherine, and the Editorial Advisory Board of the *Tufts University Diet & Nutrition Letter. The Tufts University Guide to Total Nutrition.* HarperPerennial, 1990

Hess, Mary Abbott, M.S., R.D., Hunt, Anne Elise, and Stone, Barbara Motenko. *A Healthy Head Start.* Henry Holt & Co., 1990

Jablow, Martha M., and The Children's Hospital of Philadelphia. *A Parent's Guide to Eating Disorders and Obesity.* Delta, 1992

Jacobson, Michael F., Ph.D., and Maxwell, Bruce. *What Are We Feeding Our Kids?* Workman Publishing, 1994

Kleinman, Ronald E., M.D., Jellinek, Michael S., M.D., and Houston, Julie. *What Should I Feed My Kids?* Fawcett Columbine, 1994

LaForge, Ann E. *Tantrums: Secrets to Calming the Storm.* Pocket Books, 1996

Leach, Penelope. *Your Baby & Child from Birth to Age Five.* Alfred A. Knopf, 1990

Levenstein, Harvey. *Paradox of Plenty: A Social History of Eating in Modern America.* Oxford University Press, 1993

Moore, Carolyn E., Ph.D., R.D., Schulman, Robert, M.D., and Kerr, Mimi. *Keys to Children's Nutrition.* Barrons, 1991

Nathanson, Laura Walther, M.D., F.A.A.P. *Kidshapes: A Guide to Helping Your Children Control Their Weight.* Harper Collins, 1995

Ornish, Dean, M.D. *Dr. Dean Ornish's Program for Reversing Heart Disease.* Ballantine Books, 1990

Powter, Susan. *Stop the Insanity!* Simon & Schuster, 1993

Satter, Ellyn, R.D., M.S., C.I.C.S.W., B.C.D. *Child of Mine: Feeding with Love and Good Sense.* Bull Publishing, 1991

Satter, Ellyn, R.D., M.S., C.I.C.S.W., B.C.D. *How to*

Get Your Kid to Eat . . . But Not Too Much. Bull Publishing, 1987

Schmitt, Barton D., M.D., F.A.A.P. *Your Child's Health.* Bantam Books, 1991

Schwartzman, Michael, Ph.D., and Sachs, Judith. *The Anxious Parent.* Simon & Schuster, 1990

Spock, Benjamin, M.D., and Rothenberg, Michael B., M.D. *Dr. Spock's Baby and Child Care.* Pocket Books, 1985

Stacey, Michelle. *Consumed: Why Americans Love, Hate and Fear Food.* Simon & Schuster, 1994

Wallace, Carol McD. *Elbows off the Table, Napkin in the Lap, No Video Games during Dinner.* St. Martin's Griffin, 1996

Webb, Denise, Ph.D., R.D. *Every Mother's Survival Guide to Feeding Infants and Children.* Bantam Books, 1995

Windell, James, M.A. *Children Who Say No When You Want Them to Say Yes.* Macmillan, 1996

Windell, James, M.A. *Discipline: A Sourcebook of 50 Failsafe Techniques for Parents.* Collier Books, 1991

ARTICLES

Carlton, Susan. "Living with Food Allergies." *Parents,* August, 1995

Diamond, Deborah. "Restaurant Nightmares You Can Avoid." *Parents,* August, 1995

Hagan, Carolyn. "A Get-Well Guide to Tummy Aches." *Child,* December/January, 1996

Hales, Dianne. "How to Help Your Kids Grow Up Loving Food." *Parade,* November 12, 1995

Herman, Mindy, R.D. " 'Help! My Child Hates Meat.' " *Child,* March, 1994

Herman, Mindy, R.D. "Tips from the Tooth Fairy." *Child,* June/July, 1994

Herman, Mindy, R.D. "8 Nutrition Myths Even Smart Parents Believe." *Child,* December/January, 1995

Herman, Mindy, R.D. "Raising a Fruit and Veggie Lover." *Child,* June/July 1995

Kutner, Lawrence, Ph.D. "Too fat? Too Thin?" *Parents,* July 1995

Laliberte, Richard. "How Safe Is Your Child's Food?" *Parents,* May, 1995

Leach, Penelope, Ph.D. "Help Your Child Eat Healthy Now . . . and Avoid Food Hang-ups Later." *Child,* August, 1995

McDonough, Lisa Conners. "Food Allergy Alert." *Child,* February, 1993

McDonough, Lisa Conners. "Power Snacks: Why Kids Need to Nibble." *Child,* April, 1993

Meltsner, Susan. "The New Skinny on Overweight Kids." *Child,* September, 1996

Munson, Marty, with Smith, Susan C. "Get Your Kids to Eat Right." *Prevention,* March, 1995

O'Neill, Molly. "The Morality of Fat." *The New York Times Magazine,* March 10, 1996

Prose, Francine. "The Covert Vegetable." *Parents,* April, 1993

Satter, Ellyn, R.D., M.S.W., with Israeloff, Roberta. "Picky, Picky, Picky." *Parents,* January, 1994

Siegel, Paula. " 'I Won't Eat That!' " *Redbook,* March, 1995

Stern, Loraine, M.D. "Pizza for Breakfast?" *Woman's Day,* February 21, 1995

Toscano, Siobhan Fergus. "Lovin' Spoonfuls." *Parents,* April, 1995

Weissbourd, Bernice. "How to Live With a Picky Eater." *Parents,* October, 1988

Weissbourd, Bernice. "Picky Eaters." *Parents,* January, 1991

Wood, Stephanie. "Starting Solids Step by Step." *Child,* April, 1996

Wood, Stephanie. "Moving on to Finger Foods." *Child,* April, 1996

Wood, Stephanie. "The Fluid Factor." *Child,* April, 1996

BOOKLETS

"Nutrition and Your Health: Dietary Guidelines for Americans." Fourth Edition. Published by the U.S. Department of Agriculture and the U.S. Department of Health and Human Services, 1995

ORGANIZATIONS

For more information on feeding children, or for referrals to experts who specialize in children and eating, contact the:

American Academy of Pediatrics
141 Northwest Point Blvd.
P.O. Box 927
Elk Grove Village, IL 60009-0927
(800) 433-9016

American Dietetic Association
National Center for Nutrition and Dietetics
216 West Jackson Blvd.
Chicago, IL 60606-6995
(800) 366-1655

American Heart Association
National Center
7272 Greenville Avenue
Dallas, TX 75231-4596
(800) AHA-USA1

Center for Science in the Public Interest
1875 Connecticut Avenue NW
Suite 300
Washington, DC 20009-5728
(202) 332-9110

Human Nutrition Information Service
Room 325A
Federal Building
Hyattsville, MD 29782
(301) 436-7725

Children's Nutrition Research Center
Baylor College of Medicine
1100 Bates St.
Houston, TX 77030-2600
(713) 798-7002

ALSO OF INTEREST

Menu for Mealtimes, an annotated list of stories and
   activities to teach nutrition to children. Send $4 to:
   Children's Services Department, Middle Country
   Public Library, 101 Eastwood Blvd., Centereach,
   NY 11720-2745
Tiny Tummies Nutrition News newsletter. Send $24 for
   one-year subscription to: Tiny Tummies, P.O. Box
   2171, Sausalito, CA 94966-2171, or call (415)
   389-6494

About the Author

Ann E. LaForge is a contributing editor at *Child* Magazine. She has written hundreds of articles on children, health, parenting, psychology, and other topics for numerous national publications, including *The New York Times, Child, Redbook, Good Housekeeping,* and *Healthy Kids*. She is also author of the book *Tantrums: Secrets to Calming the Storm,* and the mother of two wild but wonderful sons, who would always rather eat their dessert first.

child

The magazine for today's parents

New solutions, fresh ideas, expert advice, good old common sense and the experiences of people like you who are raising kids in the real world. Read it first in child.

YES!

Send me a free issue of child.

If I like it I'll receive a one year subscription (10 issues in all, including my free issue) for just $8.97 — a savings of over 69% off newsstand. If I choose not to subscribe, I simply return the bill marked "cancel." The free issue is mine to keep.

To order call 1-800-777-0222 extension 1122
Rate good in U.S. only

....

Look for all the helpful books in the child magazine series

**POCKET
BOOKS**

SLEEP
TANTRUMS
GOODBYES
EATING
QUARRELING
WHINING

1220-01

Having Your Baby...

...Raising Your Child

○ **BABY NAMES FROM AROUND THE WORLD**
MAXINE FIELDS
72760-5/$5.99

○ **DR. SPOCK'S BABY AND CHILD CARE**
BENJAMIN SPOCK, M.D. AND MICHAEL ROTHENBERG,M.D.
76060-2/$7.99

○ **WHAT SHALL WE NAME THE BABY?**
EDITED BY WINTHROP AMES
70962-3/$5.99

○ **BOY OR GIRL?**
DR. ELIZABETH WHELAN
73901-8/$5.99

○ **NURSING YOUR BABY**
KAREN PRYOR
4548-4/$6.99

○ **TOILET TRAINING IN LESS THAN A DAY**
DR. NATHAN AZRI & DR. RICHARD M. FOXX
69380-8/$5.99

Available from Pocket Books